HOW LIFE BEGINS
A Look at Birth and Care in the Animal World

HOW LIFE BEGINS

A Look at Birth and Care
in the Animal World

photographs by
Oxford Scientific Films

text by
Chrissy Rankin

in conjunction with
Jennifer Coldrey

G. P. PUTNAM'S SONS   NEW YORK

First American edition, 1985.
Text copyright © 1984 by Chrissy Rankin
Photographs copyright © 1984 by Oxford Scientific Films
All rights reserved.
Printed in Hong Kong by South China Printing Co.
Library of Congress Cataloging in Publication Data
Rankin, Chrissy.
How life begins.
1. Reproduction—Juvenile literature.
2. Parental behavior in animals—Juvenile literature.
3. Animals, Infancy of—Juvenile literature.
I. Oxford Scientific Films. II. Title.
QP251.5.R36   1985   591.1'6   84-42786
ISBN 0-399-21199-3
G. P. Putnam's Sons, 51 Madison Avenue, NYC 10010
First impression

Introduction

Human birth is such an intensely personal experience, and parenting is surrounded by so much theory and anxiety, that it is easy for humans to think of themselves as different and superior to the rest of creation. In fact, we differ from other mammals only in consciousness, and it is easy for adults to give children the impression that "animals" are less sensitive, less caring, and more nonchalant in the treatment of their young than "civilized" human beings.

But animals do "care" about the welfare of their young, even though this care may be instinctive. And the attitudes of most human parents to their newborn baby are largely instinctive, whatever the cultural or sociological fashion.

This book shows the lengths to which animals will go to ensure the survival of their kind. They may shed millions of eggs into water, and perhaps two eggs will survive. They may lay their eggs on a food supply so that the newly hatched larvae are supplied with nourishment. They may construct a nest in which their eggs are incubated and in which the young creatures are cared for until ready to leave. Or they may give birth to a single, live youngster which is carefully nurtured.

By shedding light on some of the fascinating and complex ways in which parental care is exercised, whether before or after birth, this book, with its stunning pictures and informative text, should increase children's respect for animals.

Contents

Reproduction

Eggs

Live birth

Parental care

Reproduction

Very simple ways of reproducing

All living creatures reproduce, but they do so in different ways. Some very tiny animals, like amoebas, simply divide into two parts. They do not need a partner. After they have divided, each part lives a separate existence and in time it also divides into two parts. This method of reproduction allows these small creatures to increase their numbers very quickly.

Other small animals, like hydras, creatures related to jellyfish and sea anemones, reproduce by budding. A bud or bump forms on the body and grows into a new hydra. When the bud is fully formed, but still small, it breaks away to become independent.

Division and budding are both forms of reproduction where no partner is needed. Animals that reproduce in this way always have young exactly like themselves.

Larger animals are more complicated and they cannot multiply by simply splitting into new individuals. These animals have had to find a different way of reproducing.

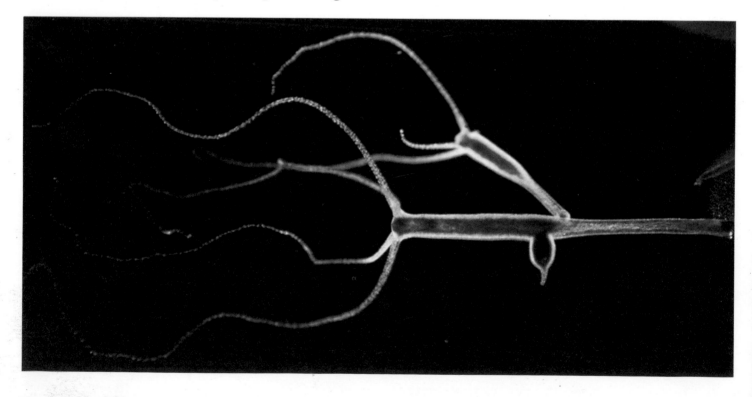

Hydra budding

This freshwater hydra, which is about $\frac{2}{5}$ in. long, is reproducing by budding. Two buds have formed on the side of the parent's body. One is still young. The other has grown tentacles and is nearly ready to break off and start life on its own.

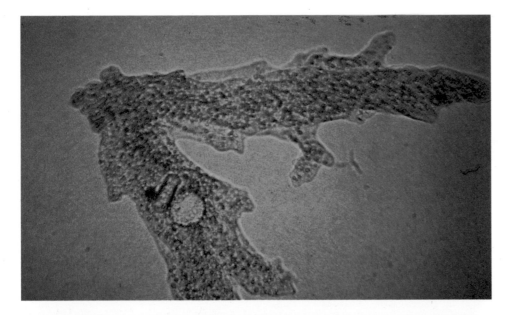

Amoeba dividing

An amoeba is a very tiny creature that can be seen only through a microscope. It reproduces by dividing into two. Here the division is nearly complete and each half will eventually move apart to live on its own. When each part grows to full size it will divide again.

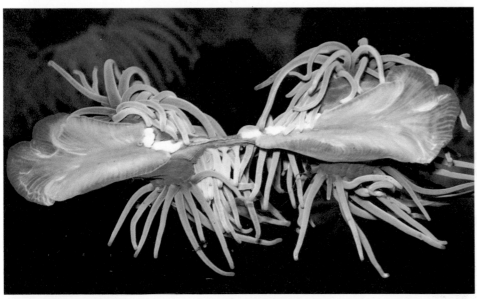

Snakelocks sea anemone dividing

Sea anemones can reproduce in several different ways. This snake-locks sea anemone is dividing into two. It splits down the middle from tentacles to base. The two parts have nearly separated and each will form a new animal.

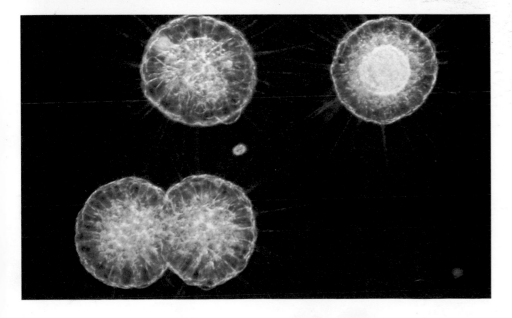

Sun animals

Sun animals, like amoebas, are very tiny creatures found in peaty pools. They are rarely more than $\frac{1}{25}$ in. across. Also like amoebas they reproduce by dividing into two. In this picture are three sun animals, one of which is beginning to divide into two creatures.

The need for two parents

Most living things have two parents—a male and a female. This is true of plants, animals and people.

Male and female bodies are different because during reproduction they have different jobs to do. The female produces tiny egg cells which contain information from the mother. The male produces sperm cells which are much smaller than the egg and contain information from the father. Eggs and sperm are called sex cells and are produced in a special place inside each parent's body.

Before a young animal can be born a male and female must mate. During mating the male and female come together so eggs and sperm can join. When they have joined together, an egg cell is said to be "fertilized." Now the young animal or "embryo" will start to grow. Because the young animal develops from both the sperm and egg it will be partly like its mother and partly like its father—but different from both.

For many animals that live in the water, mating is fairly simple. The parents come close together and millions of sperm and eggs are released into the water at the same time. The sperm swim through the water and join with the eggs. Any egg that becomes fertilized can then start to grow.

Brown trout
Here the male brown trout is swimming close to the female during mating. The female lays her eggs on the bed of a shallow river. As the eggs are released the male sheds his sperm over them. Sperm can swim only a short distance, so the parents have to make sure they are close to each other to mate.

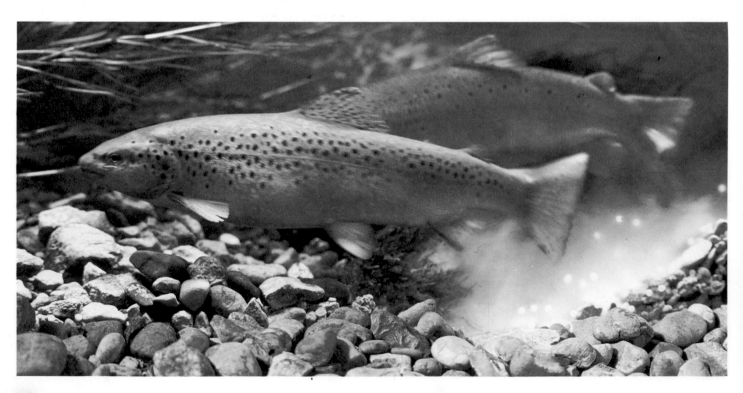

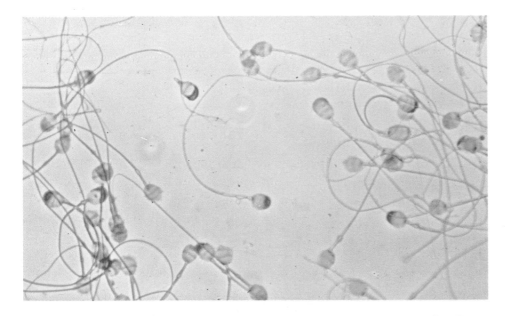

Sperm

When seen through a powerful microscope most sperm look like tiny tadpoles. In this picture, mouse sperm have been magnified over 1000 times. We can see that each one has a long tail which it waves to and fro to help it swim toward the egg. The egg is round and much larger than the sperm. It hardly moves at all.

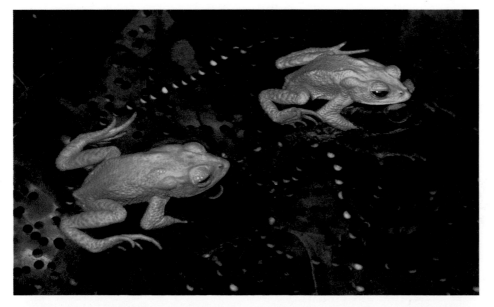

Golden toads

Like most frogs and toads, these golden toads mate in water. The male clings tightly to the female's back during mating. His sexual opening, from which the sperm are shed, is then brought close to the female's. As her long string of eggs is laid, the sperm flows over them and fertilization takes place.

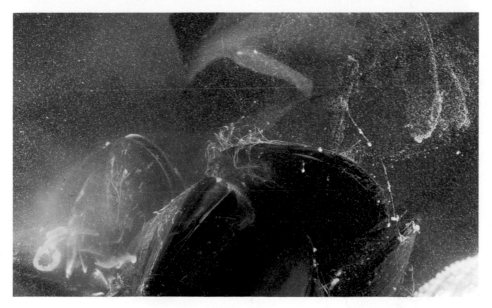

Mussels

Animals like these mussels are attached to one spot during their adult life and cannot move to-gether to mate. They make sure their sex cells are shed into the water at the same time by reacting to an outside signal. Mussels respond to the warmth of the water around them. When the water reaches a certain tem-perature, a milky cloud of sperm and a mass of eggs are shed into the water at the same time.

The need for two parents
continued

When eggs and sperm join together outside a female's body many eggs never become fertilized. Another way of mating is for the male to place the sperm inside the female's body near to her "ovaries," where the eggs are produced. The sperm are then more sure of reaching the eggs which become fertilized before they are laid. This way of mating is essential when animals live on land, as there is no water to carry the sperm to the eggs.

A few animals that live in water mate in this way. Octopus and squid shed their sperm in small packets which are placed inside the female during mating. Male sharks have two special fins on the underside of their body. These are held together during mating to form a tube and through this tube the male's sperm enters the female's opening.

Birds mate in a different way. Their sexual openings are under their tails. During mating the male balances on top of the female's back, steadying himself with his beak. He then twists his tail so that his sexual opening can join with hers. Millions of sperm, carried in a liquid, are then passed from the male to the female.

Some animals have a special organ for passing sperm into the female's body. In male snakes, lizards, a few birds and all mammals, including man, this organ is called a penis. During mating the penis is placed inside the female's opening and the sperm are released through it. Most male insects also have a special organ for depositing sperm inside the female.

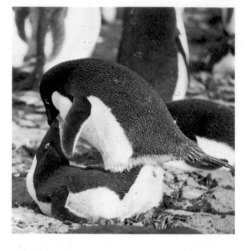

Penguins
Female penguins, like other birds, have to keep very still during mating, so that the male does not lose his balance and topple off! A long winding tube called the "oviduct" leads from the opening below the female's tail to the ovary. After mating the male's sperm swim up the oviduct to fertilize the eggs.

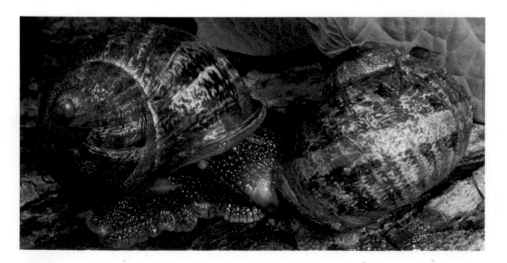

Snails mating
Not all animals have separate males and females. In earthworms, slugs and snails, each animal is both male and female and can produce both sperm and eggs. These are called "hermaphrodite" animals. They mate in pairs so that they can exchange their sperm to fertilize each other's eggs.

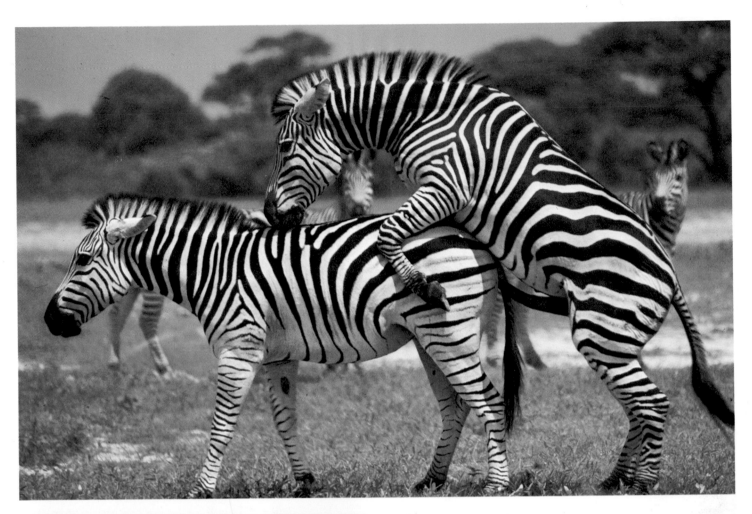

Zebra

Most mammals, like this zebra, use the piggyback position for mating. The male mounts on top of the female so that his penis can enter the female's opening.

Butterflies

These common blue butterflies face in opposite directions while they mate. In this way their rear ends are joined together while the male deposits his sperm inside the female.

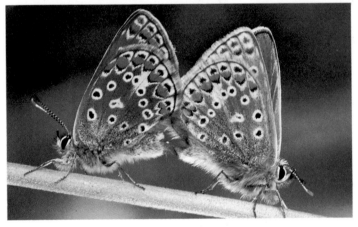

House spiders

A few days before mating the male house spider, which is smaller than the female, spins a small web into which he places a drop of sperm. He then stores the sperm packet in a pair of short legs, called palps, near to his mouth, and goes in search of a female. During mating the palps are placed inside the female's sexual opening and the packet is released. The silken web dissolves and the sperm are free to swim to the eggs.

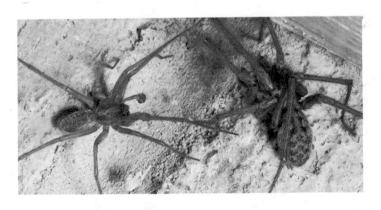

Eggs
Animals that lay eggs

When you think of an egg you probably think of the smooth, hard-shelled eggs of birds. But many other animals lay eggs. In water, crabs, jellyfish, corals, sea urchins, octopus, frogs and most fish lay eggs. On land, the egg-laying animals include insects, spiders and snails, many reptiles and, of course, birds. There are also two mammals, the duck-billed platypus and the spiny anteater, that lay eggs, (see page 57).

Eggs laid in water are in no danger of drying out and so do not need thick protective shells. Animals that lay their eggs on land, however, have to prevent them from losing water. They do this by surrounding each egg with a thick shell which is very nearly watertight. Fertilization has to take place before the shell is formed as the shell would prevent any sperm from reaching the egg. Inside the shell the embryo develops in safety until it is ready to hatch.

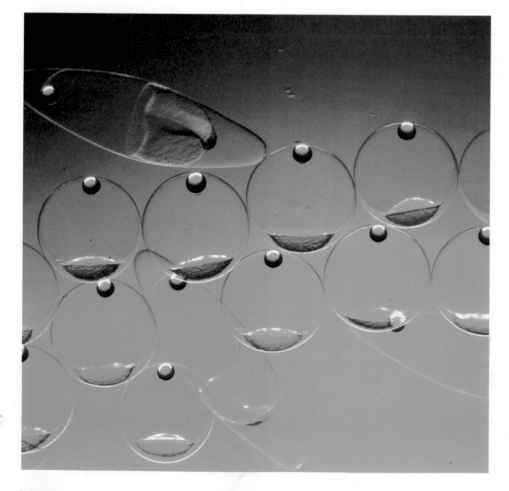

Fish eggs
These tiny fish eggs, like those of many other sea creatures, float in the water. Inside each egg is a drop of oil which makes the eggs rise close to the water's surface. Here, where there is warmth and plenty of oxygen, they drift with the ocean currents and the young start to grow.

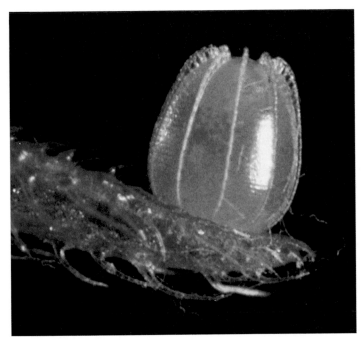

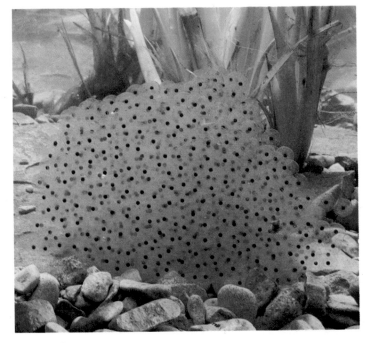

Insect eggs

The eggs of insects come in many shapes and sizes and may be laid singly or in groups. Eggs laid in open places where they are exposed to wind and rain have thick shells. Those hidden underground or in other sheltered places have thin shells. The eggs of the comma butterfly have thick shells and are laid singly on nettle leaves. The eggs are oval-shaped, hard and about the size of a pin head.

Frogs' eggs

Amphibians (frogs, toads, newts, etc.), and some insects like the dragonfly and mosquito that spend their adult life on land have to return to water to lay their eggs. Their eggs have no protective shells and if laid on land would quickly dry out. Frogs lay large masses of eggs which we call frog-spawn. Each egg is surrounded in jelly which swells in water and allows the eggs to float. The eggs stick together in a great mass, which makes it difficult and unpleasant for hungry animals to eat them.

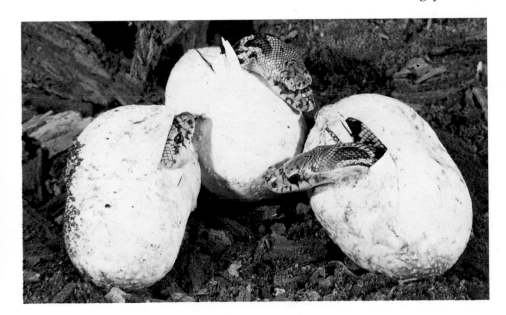

Snakes' eggs

Reptiles, such as snakes, lizards and turtles, lay eggs with soft, leathery shells. During development the egg absorbs water and it swells until the shell becomes very tight. Just before hatching young snakes grow a sharp tooth, called an egg-tooth, on their snouts. As each youngster twists and turns, to try to get out of its egg, the tooth slits the shell in several places. Through one of these holes the young snake escapes. The egg-tooth drops off soon after hatching.

Growing within an egg

After fertilization the egg cell of a hen starts its journey down the female's oviduct. During this journey various layers are formed.

The first layer is the yellow yolk—a large ball of food to nourish the growing young. Formed around the yolk and egg cell is a layer of white, a clear jellylike layer, which is a mixture of food and water. Each of these two layers has a thin transparent skin around it. The final layer is the shell which surrounds all these soft inner parts. When the shell has hardened, the hen's egg is ready to be laid. At the broad end of the egg, between the white and the shell, is an airspace.

After it has been laid, the fertilized egg cell inside the shell begins to divide. It divides over and over again until all the different cells of the new chick are formed. During development tiny blood vessels spread over the yolk and white and to the airspace. The blood takes in food from the yolk and white, and oxygen from the airspace, and carries them to the developing embryo. Both oxygen and food are needed for the young chick to develop.

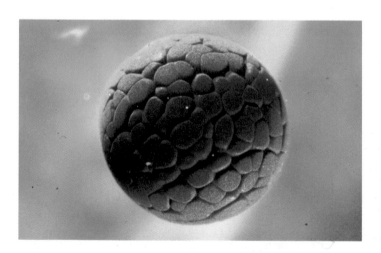

Frogs' egg dividing
Frogs' eggs float near the surface of the water where they are warmed by the heat of the sun. During the first two days, after the egg has been fertilized, each egg cell divides over and over again. These divisions are too small to be seen unless the egg is looked at through a microscope, which is how this photograph has been taken.

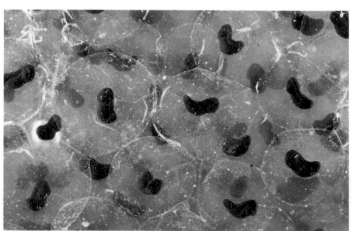

Developing frogs' embryos
After two days the ball of cells begins to lengthen and a head and tail can be seen. The developing frogs' embryos feed on the yolk in the same way as growing birds do. Ten days after being laid the jelly turns to liquid and the tadpoles wriggle free. For the next few days they feed on the remains of the yolk until their mouths are fully developed.

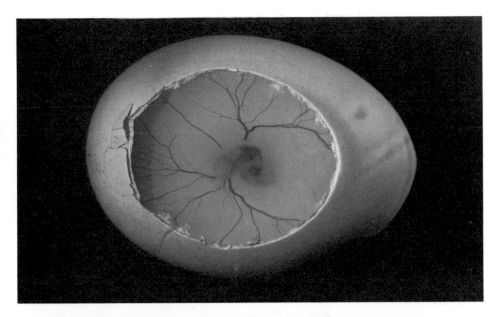

Chick embryo

The developing chick embryo after $3\frac{1}{2}$–4 days is still only a speck on the egg yolk. But it already has a head and a backbone and the eyes are beginning to develop. Notice the blood vessels spreading over the yellow yolk. These carry food, oxygen and water to the growing embryo.

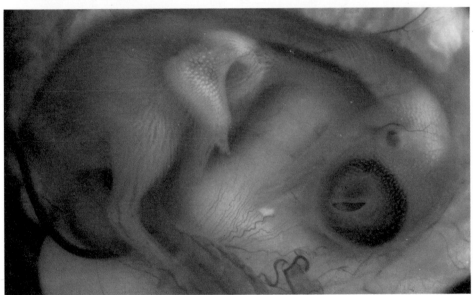

After 12 days the chick embryo is beginning to look more like a small bird. It is feathered and has well-developed eyes and a brain. Like young reptiles the chick has an egg-tooth on its beak. This helps it to hatch from the egg.

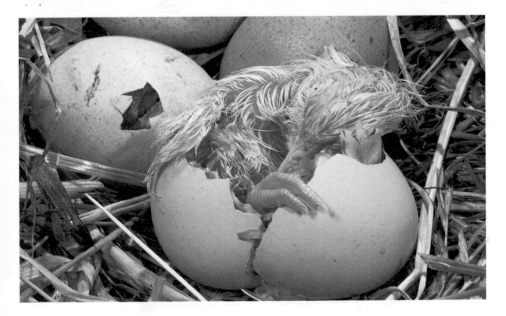

Chick hatching

After three weeks the chick is fully formed, filling the egg and ready to hatch. Using its egg-tooth it pecks at the shell until it is able to break out. When it first comes out of the egg the chick is tired, weak and wet, but it soon dries out and starts to run around and peck for food. After 24 hours the egg-tooth drops off.

Water larvae

The embryo growing within the egg feeds on the yolk. If there is a large store of yolk, as in bird and reptile eggs, then the embryo can grow quite big and is well developed before hatching.

The eggs of many animals, especially those that live in water, are very small and have only a little yolk. The young hatch quickly as the yolk is soon used up and they need to find more food. When these youngsters hatch they usually look quite unlike their parents, both in size and shape. They are called "larvae."

Larvae change their shape and form at least once before they become adults. Their lives are often completely different from their parents. The larvae of many sea creatures, for example mussels, shrimps and sponges, float near the water's surface feeding on tiny plants. Many of them are so small they can be seen clearly only under a microscope. They are delicate, often transparent, creatures which makes them almost invisible to hungry enemies (called "predators").

Not all water larvae are microscopic floating creatures. Some that hatch and grow in freshwater, like the tadpole of a frog, are quite big and very active.

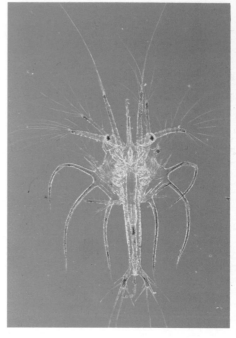

Shrimp larva
This strange transparent animal is the larva of a shrimp and is only $\frac{2}{25}$ in. long. The tough spiky horns sticking out from its body help it to float in the sea and also protect it from being eaten. A larva like this will eventually grow too big and heavy to float and will gradually sink to the bottom of the sea. Here it will change into the adult form.

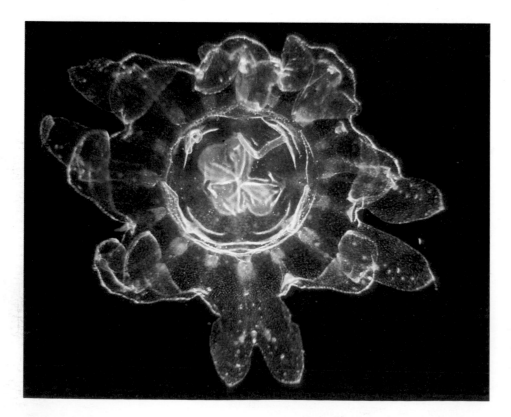

Jellyfish larva
Some larvae are very beautiful and look like tiny floating flowers, as this young jellyfish does. Now only $\frac{2}{5}$ in. wide, this larva will one day grow into an adult jellyfish about 10 in. across.

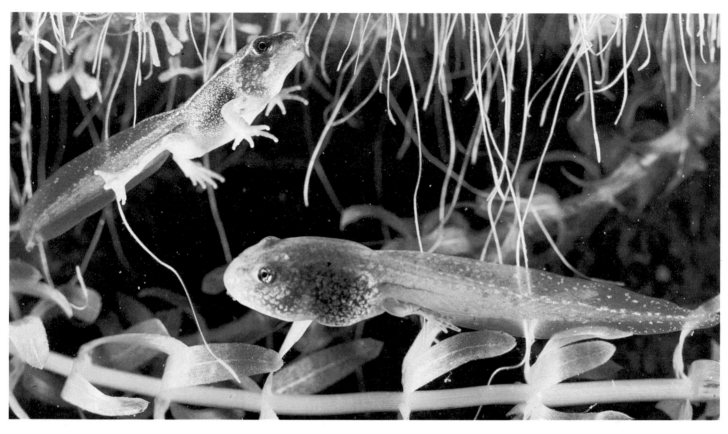

Tadpoles

Tadpoles of the common frog live in freshwater where they first feed on weeds and then later on small animals such as insects and worms. During their life in the water many tadpoles are eaten by other animals such as fish and birds. About seven weeks after hatching a tadpole begins to grow back legs. At 13 weeks it has developed into a froglet, having grown both back and front legs and lost its tail. Three weeks later the small frogs leave the water and hop off to explore their new home on land.

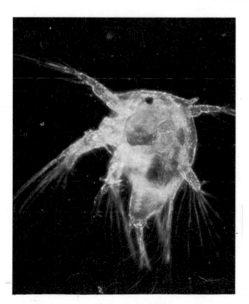

Barnacle larva

Many water larvae are carried far away from their parents by tides and currents. This is very important for animals like mussels and barnacles, which are fixed to rocks or the seabed during their adult life. Like this barnacle larva, the young are carried away from the over-crowded homes of their parents. They will find new places to live and will not have to compete with the stronger adults for food and space.

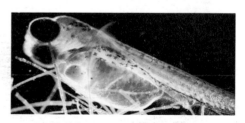

Young stickleback

Looking rather like an adult fish in shape, this newly hatched stickleback is hiding among weeds for safety. For the first few days after hatching it feeds from the large yolk sac on its belly. When all the yolk is finished it feeds on tiny animals in the water around it.

Land larvae

On land there are also young animals that hatch from the egg as larvae. The commonest are the larvae of insects, like the caterpillars of moths and butterflies, the grubs of beetles and the maggots of flies. These larvae look quite different from their parents and have to pass through several stages before becoming adults. The young of grasshoppers, earwigs and cockroaches, however, look similar to their parents but are smaller and dumpier with no wings. These young are called "nymphs."

As young insects grow bigger their skins become tight. It is now time to "molt." A new skin forms beneath the old one, which then splits apart. Out wriggles the larva or nymph in its new soft coat which then hardens. All insect young molt several times during their larval stage. Some, like caterpillar and ladybird larvae, then go through one more stage before becoming an adult. At their final molt their skin splits to reveal a hard-shelled object—the "pupa." Inside the pupa the larva's body gradually changes into the adult insect.

Many insects like dragonflies, mayflies and some butterflies spend nearly all their life as larvae and live as adults only for a very short time, just long enough to mate and lay eggs.

Caterpillar hatching
Inside a butterfly's egg the embryo grows and finally hatches as a small caterpillar. These young cabbage white caterpillars are biting their way out of their eggs. Once free they will eat the egg shell, which provides them with essential food before they start to feed on cabbage leaves.

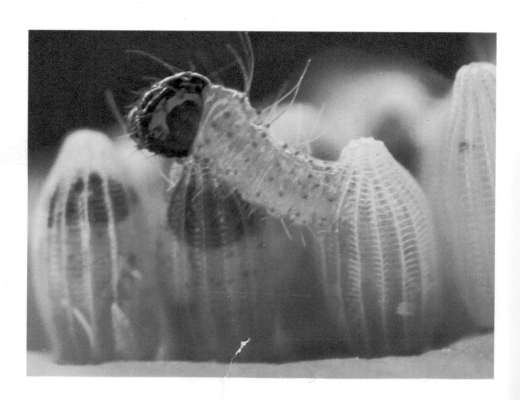

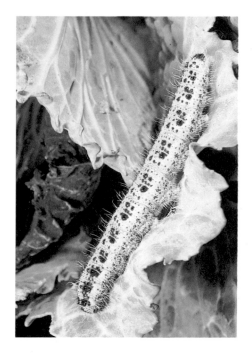

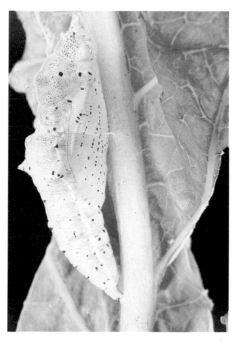

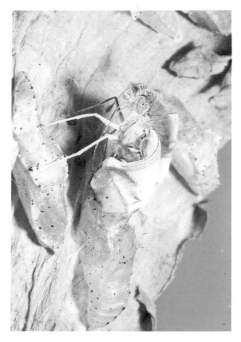

Caterpillar

The caterpillar is a hungry creature and feeds on many juicy cabbage leaves. It grows rapidly and molts several times before reaching its full size. This may take several weeks. When the caterpillar reaches full size it stops eating and is ready to change into a pupa.

Pupa

Each cabbage white caterpillar now moves to a dry, sheltered place to pupate. It attaches itself to a leaf with a silken thread and is held firm at the bottom by a silken pad. Moth caterpillars often surround themselves in a cocoon of silk. At the last molt the larva turns into a pupa. At first the pupa is soft and pale but it soon darkens and hardens.

The butterfly appears

Many insects spend several weeks or maybe months in the pupal stage. The cabbage white butterfly emerges after only 2–3 weeks, by which time the cabbage leaf has withered and turned brown. Here the pupal skin has split and the adult butterfly is pulling itself out. At first it looks rather crumpled but will hang upside down and pump blood into its wings until they expand and harden. The butterfly is then ready to fly off to feed and then to mate.

Cockroach and young

Cockroach nymphs look very like the adults but without the wings. At their final molt, ten months to one year after hatching, the adult emerges with its wings fully formed. The young are white when they hatch from the egg and for a short while after each molt, but they soon harden and turn brown. Both nymphs and adults feed on the same sort of food.

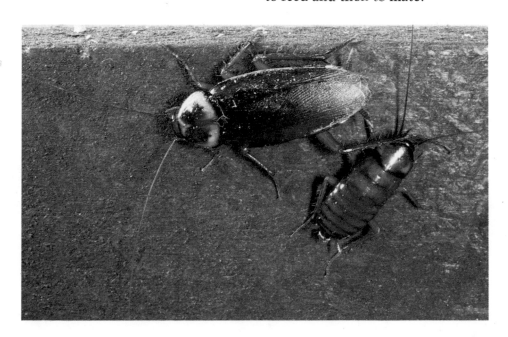

Mass production in the sea

Most animals that live and breed in the sea lay their eggs and then leave them. When the young hatch they have to look after themselves. Jellyfish, starfish, some sea urchins and many fish leave their eggs in this way.

Many of these eggs are not fertilized. Those that are, float to the surface of the sea where they hatch into tiny larvae. The surface of the sea is like a gigantic nursery, full of hundreds of different kinds of young animals, all feeding and growing together. It is also a very dangerous place, full of hungry creatures ready to eat both eggs and young. Although many young are protected to some extent by being transparent and invisible, their chances of survival are very small.

The young of sponges, sea anemones and other animals that are fixed to one spot during their adult life face other hazards. Only those that sink to the sea bottom and land on rocks and stones will survive, because there they are able to anchor themselves and continue growing. Many land on sand, seaweed and other unsuitable places and are likely to die.

Animals that leave their young lay huge numbers of eggs at a time. This ensures that at least a few will survive. A female cod lays as many as 5 million eggs, of which perhaps only two will survive to adulthood. Starfish can lay $2\frac{1}{2}$ million eggs, while mussels release 5–12 million eggs at a time.

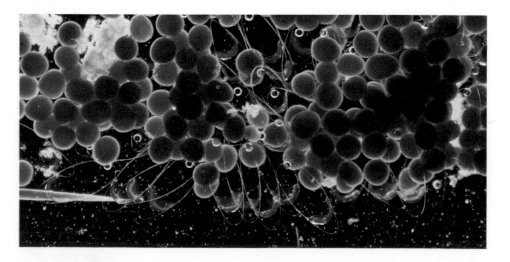

Egg mass
Mingled together in this drop of seawater are a mass of fish eggs and sponge larvae. The oval-shaped sponge larvae are solid creatures and not at all transparent. They are covered with tiny beating hairs which help to hold them up in the water. These larvae float in the water for about 24 hours before sinking to the sea-bottom to grow into adults.

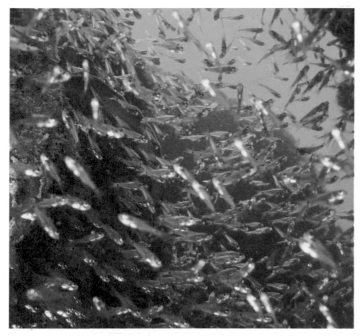

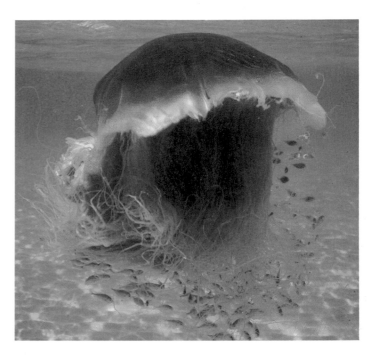

Young fish

Many young fish like these live together in huge groups for protection. The large numbers swimming closely together help to confuse any hunter about to attack. The hunter finds it difficult to chase an individual fish. If it does attack, the group quickly splits and scatters.

Jellyfish and small fish

Some young animals have found amazing ways to protect themselves from the dangers of the sea. Seeking shelter under the umbrellas of giant jellyfish, these young fish remain safe for a while. Unlike most creatures, they are not hurt by the jellyfish's poisonous tentacles. Other creatures do not try to eat them as they are afraid of being stung by the jellyfish.

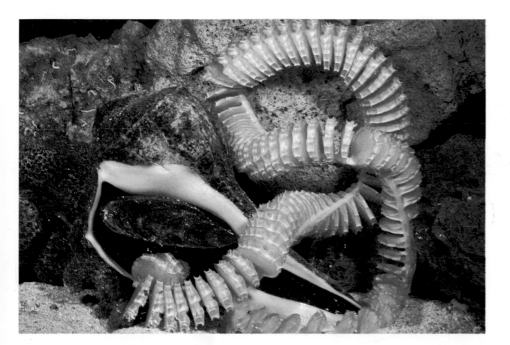

Atlantic whelk

The egg capsules of the Atlantic whelk, a type of sea snail, are laid in a long string. Each capsule can have up to 100 eggs in it. Of these only a dozen or so hatch. The rest provide a store of food for the developing young. The young complete their larval stage within the capsule and hatch as miniature copies of their parents.

Freshwater animals that leave their eggs

Many freshwater animals also lay their eggs and then leave them. Freshwater animals lay fewer eggs than sea creatures, and they usually leave them in safe places. One of the dangers of laying eggs in streams and rivers is that they can easily be washed downstream.

The female toad lays her eggs in long strings which she wraps around waterplants and stones for safety. Dragonflies and mayflies may attach their eggs to waterplants, while many fish hide their eggs under pebbles on the riverbed. The female brown trout forms a shallow groove on the riverbed by lying on her side and flapping her tail to move aside the sand and gravel. Into the groove she lays her eggs, which become buried under the sand and remain safe.

Freshwater eggs have a big yolk and this allows more time for the embryo to grow within the safety of the egg. Compared to most sea creatures young freshwater animals hatch at a well-developed stage and are better able to cope with their dangerous world. The larvae of creatures like the great diving beetle and the nymph of the dragonfly are very fierce. They hunt and eat tadpoles, small fish and other small animals, but they in their turn may be eaten by larger creatures. Many larvae hide among weeds and stones for safety.

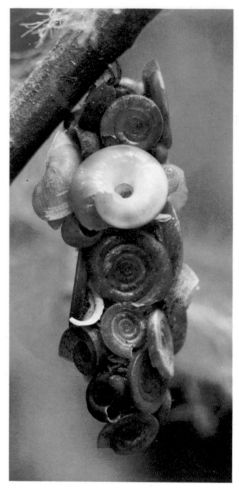

Great pond snail

The great pond snail lays its eggs in a sausage-shaped mass of jelly for protection. This is usually attached to the leaves or stem of a waterplant, but here the eggs are being laid on the glass of an aquarium. The pond snail's eggs have very large yolks, and the young are able to grow into tiny snails, complete with shells, before hatching.

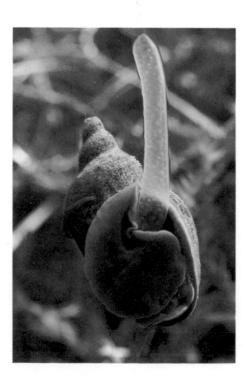

Caddis fly larva

The eggs of the caddis fly are laid during spring and summer. Some females crawl under water to lay their eggs, while others drop their eggs onto the water as they fly over the surface. The larva, on hatching, has an unusual way of protecting itself. It covers its soft body in a silken case to which it attaches small sand grains, shells, pieces of plant and other objects. The case is open at one end so that the larva can put its head and legs out to move and feed, as you can see. Within this home the larva can hide if in any danger. The heavy case also holds the larva down on the stream bed so that it doesn't float away.

Adult mosquito hatching and egg raft

Many insects lay their eggs in water. The 200–300 eggs of the mosquito float together like a raft on the surface of ponds and other still water. The larvae hatch and spend several days feeding in the water before turning into pupae. The adult mosquito finally hatches through a split in the pupal case. This takes place at the water's surface so the mosquito can climb out, stretch its wings and fly away.

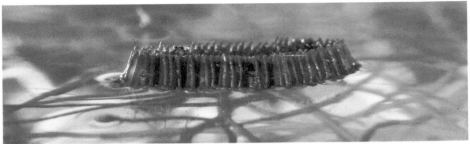

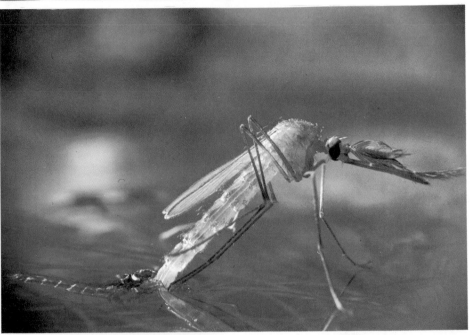

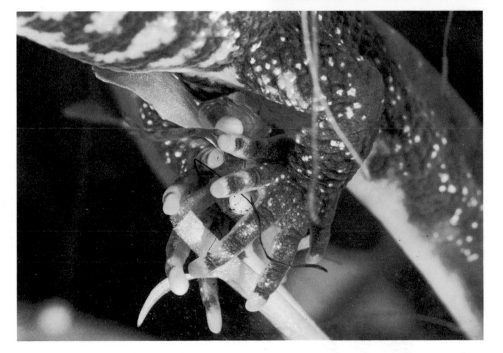

Great crested newt

The female great crested newt lays each egg singly on the leaves of waterplants. She chooses each leaf by smell and touch. Then, taking hold of the leaf with her hind feet, she folds it over to form a tube and lays an egg in it. Each egg is surrounded in jelly which glues the leaf firmly around the egg to protect it. The tadpoles hatch after 2–3 weeks.

Land animals that leave their eggs

Land animals that abandon their eggs generally lay only about 50–100 compared to the thousands or millions laid by sea creatures. The young stay within the safety of the egg until they are well developed and the youngsters that hatch are able to look after themselves right away.

Many snails, worms, insects and reptiles leave their eggs when they have laid them. But before leaving them the female often buries or hides her eggs for safety. Some spiders will wrap their eggs in a waterproof cocoon of silk before hiding them.

When a young animal hatches out of its egg the first thing it needs is food. Many of these independent young discover what to eat by trial and error. A young chameleon knows instinctively that it has to shoot out its tongue to catch insects. With a little practice it becomes a perfect shot. Baby lizards and snakes need to find insects, spiders and small frogs. Tiny spiders quickly spin a web to trap midges and flies. If these young animals do not soon learn where to find food they will grow weak and die.

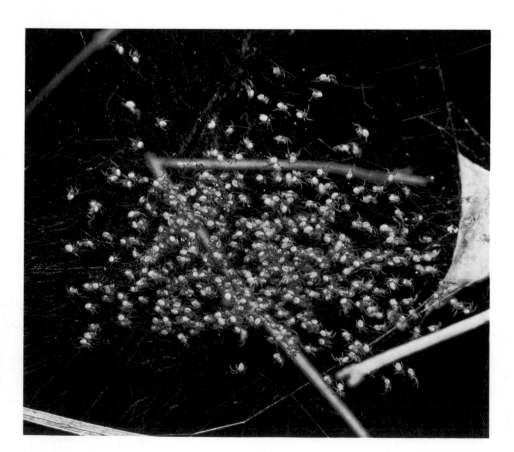

Spiderlings

Hundreds of tiny spiderlings emerge from the abandoned cocoon of an orb weaving spider. The young are hungry and separate quickly—if they stay together too long they start to eat each other! Each climbs to the top of the nearby plant, then, turning to face the breeze, it releases a long strand of silk from its abdomen. The spiderling is picked up by the wind and carried away on the silken thread to new feeding grounds.

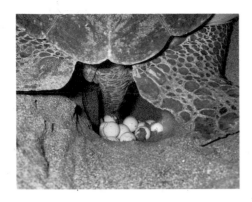

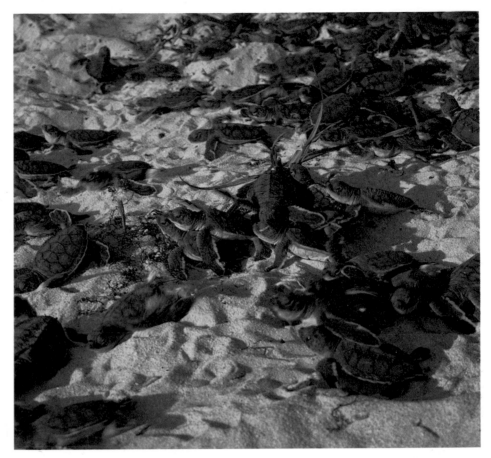

Turtle laying eggs

The female green turtle spends most of her life at sea. After mating at sea she finds a quiet sandy beach to lay her eggs at night. She digs a hole 20 in. deep with her hind flippers. Into the hole she lays 60–100 white, leathery eggs which she then covers over with sand. Before returning to the sea she shuffles over the site, disturbing the sand to hide her tracks and nest from view. The eggs are kept moist in the damp sand of the hiding place as well as being protected from hungry animals.

Young turtles

Turtle eggs take seven weeks to hatch. During this time they are warmed by the heat of the sun on the sand around them. When the young turtles hatch they dig their way up to just below the surface of the sand. As dusk falls hundreds of youngsters from many nests make a dash to the sea. This is the most dangerous journey of their lives, as many crabs and seabirds are waiting to catch and eat them. Even in the water danger awaits them. Only two or three turtles of each brood survive to become adults.

Slug laying eggs

Once the slug has laid its eggs it leaves them. Hidden among the roots of plants and under stones, they will stay safe until they hatch. Each egg is well stocked with yolk and the young grow into tiny slugs before hatching. A few weeks after the eggs have been laid the young break out and slither away.

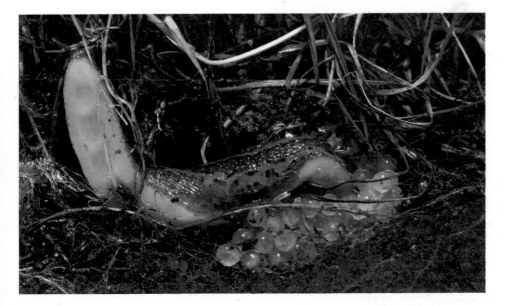

Eggs laid on a food supply

Some land animals lay their eggs on or near food that will be suitable for their young when they hatch. The young then climb out of the egg and start to feed immediately. This way of caring for the young is especially common in the insect world.

Many insects lay their eggs on the surface of the food plant. The cabbage white butterfly lays her eggs in groups on the underside of cabbage leaves. The eggs of the Colorado beetle are laid on potato leaves. Ladybugs lay their eggs near a mass of aphids.

Some larvae need to munch on food inside a plant. To help the female lay her eggs in exactly the right place she has a special egg-laying organ—the "ovipositor." Using her ovipositor, which is a long tube, the female makes a hole into the plant or animal where she can lay her eggs. The young that hatch are then surrounded by food which they can eat immediately.

The blowfly uses her ovipositor to place her eggs in the bodies of dead animals. Sawflies, as their name suggests, use their ovipositor for sawing into plant stems and leaves before laying their eggs. The giant woodwasp has an ovipositor to drill holes through the bark of pine trees and into the wood below.

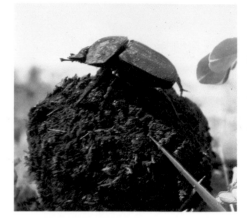

Dung beetle

African dung beetles collect the droppings of animals and roll them home to their underground chamber. There the dung is stored as a future food supply. This female is rolling a ball of elephant dung. When the time comes for her to lay eggs she collects buffalo dung and shapes it into a dozen or so balls. In each ball she lays an egg. Protected in this ball the larva hatches out and starts to eat its food supply. The larva eventually turns into a pupa inside the dung ball and emerges later as an adult beetle.

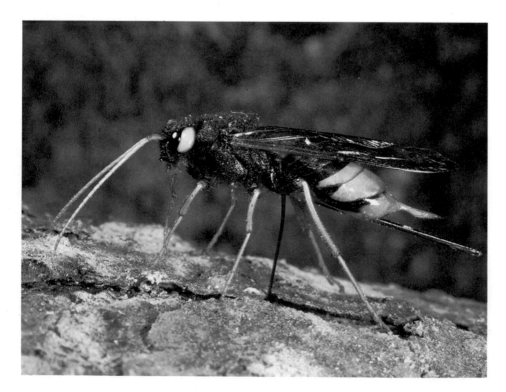

Giant woodwasp

This female woodwasp is using her long, thin, stiff ovipositor to drill a hole through the bark of a pine tree. When she reaches the soft wood beneath she lays her four or five eggs, squeezing them out of the end of her ovipositor. The eggs develop safely under the bark of the tree. When they hatch the grubs spend up to three years eating and tunneling through the wood before they turn into pupae.

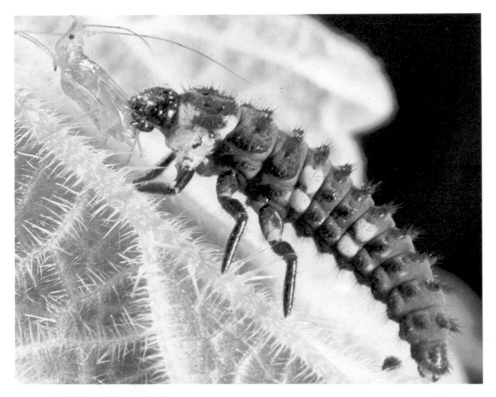

Ladybug larva with aphids

Young ladybugs feed on aphids, so the female lays her eggs in places where these tiny animals are plentiful. The young active larvae hatch 5–8 days later and quickly start hunting for food. By the time they turn into pupae they will have eaten hundreds of aphids. Ladybugs breed and lay their eggs when they are 4–7 weeks old, so that during one summer several generations may be produced.

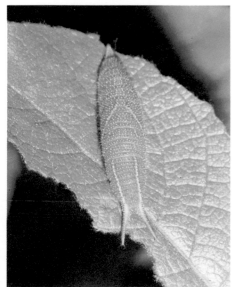

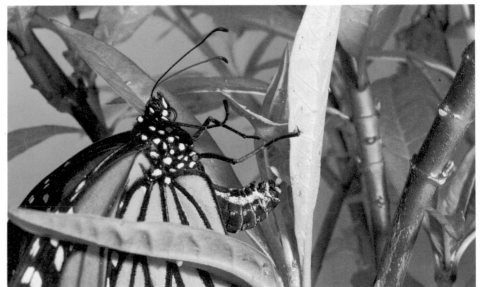

Camouflaged caterpillar

Being well "camouflaged" to look like its food plant is one way in which caterpillars hide from hungry enemies. This caterpillar of the purple emperor butterfly is exactly the same color as the sallow leaf it feeds on.

Monarch butterfly

The eggs of the monarch butterfly are laid on the leaves of the poisonous milkweed plant and take only a few days to hatch. As the caterpillars feed on the leaves and stems of the milkweed they take in its poisons with no ill effect.

But if a bird eats a caterpillar it soon becomes ill and vomits, and is unlikely to choose a monarch caterpillar again. The caterpillar's black and yellow stripes act as a warning signal.

Egg protection

Eggs are more likely to survive if they are protected by a watchful parent. In water, only a few animals, like the octopus and stickleback, guard their eggs, compared to the thousands that abandon them. Some sea animals, such as rays, skates, dogfish and whelks, lay their eggs in a thick protective case. Although the female does not stay to guard her eggs, other animals find it difficult to get through the tough casing to eat them. On land egg protection is more common. Nearly all birds watch over their eggs and also look after their young. Other animals including some spiders and insects, some frogs and a few reptiles, guard their eggs but abandon their young when they hatch. Females that look after their eggs and young usually lay fewer eggs than those that abandon them, as the chances of survival are much greater when the young are protected by their parents.

Many of these watchful parents, including several snakes and spiders, are quick to attack any hunters eager to eat their eggs. While protecting their eggs, females may have very little time to feed, and by the time the eggs hatch, the mother is weak and hungry. If the young stay near her they may be eaten!

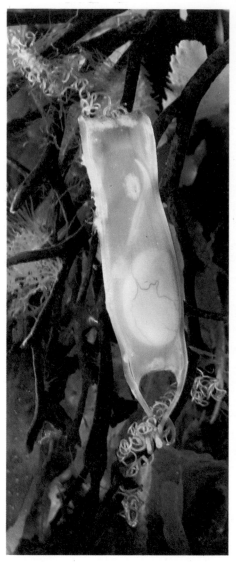

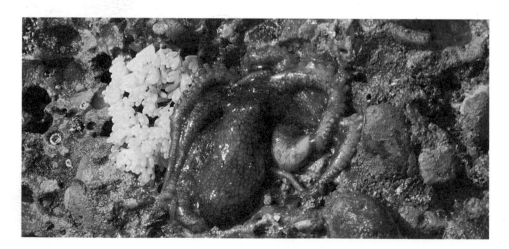

Octopus
The octopus is one of the most caring mothers. She lays her eggs in long strings which she hangs under a rock crevice and carefully guards. She cleans her eggs regularly, using her tentacle tips, and she wafts them with water so that they have a fresh supply of oxygen. Each tiny larva, on hatching, is only $\frac{1}{50}$ in. long. The larvae drift in the water for several weeks, feeding and growing and during this time many are eaten. Those that do survive sink to the seabed where they hide and eventually grow into adults.

Dogfish eggcase
The female dogfish lays only one fertilized egg inside each eggcase. A large supply of yolk fills most of the egg at first, but this gets smaller as the fish grows. At each corner of the leathery eggcase are long coiled tendrils that catch among seaweed and stop the egg being carried into deep water. Inside the eggcase the young develops in safety and after several months a fully formed fish hatches. These eggcases are called mermaid's purses and are often found empty on the beach.

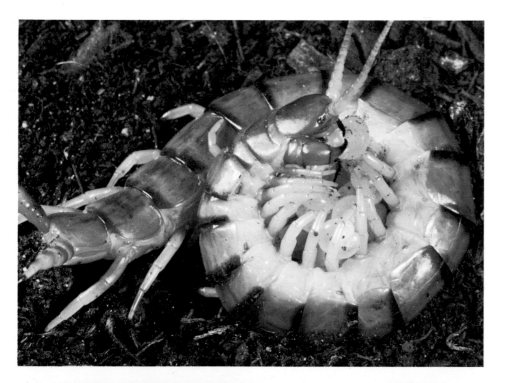

Centipede and eggs

Some centipedes are very protective toward their eggs. Here the female has coiled her body tightly around her pile of eggs. She will fight off any enemies. From time to time she uncoils herself to lick an egg, picking it up with her fangs and first pair of legs. Cleaning helps to keep the eggs free of fungus, which would kill them. If the female is disturbed however, she may abandon her eggs.

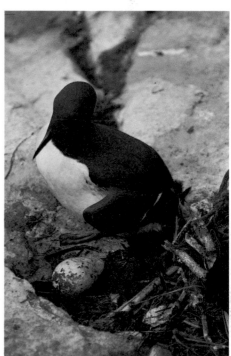

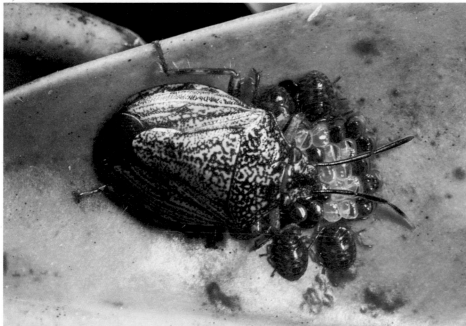

Shieldbug and brood

Like a hen brooding her eggs this shieldbug is guarding her batch of eggs and newly hatched young. The egg-mass contains about 40 eggs that are laid in a diamond-shaped cluster. It is just the right size for the female to cover with her body. After the young have hatched she will look after them for a few days before leaving them. Shieldbugs are sometimes called "parent bugs."

Colonial nesters

Seabirds like this guillemot lay their eggs on narrow ledges of sea cliffs which other animals find difficult to reach. Their eggs are pointed at one end so that if they roll they spin in a circle and do not fall off the cliff. Seabirds often nest in huge groups or "colonies." This has advantages as several birds can join together to ward off intruders eager to carry away the eggs or young.

Social insects

Some insects live together in huge colonies containing many hundreds or thousands of animals, all totally dependent on each other for their survival. Ants, termites and some bees and wasps are examples of what are called "social insects." The colony is one big family and usually all the individuals are the offspring of a single breeding female: the queen. In many colonies the queen's only job is to lay eggs. She does not feed herself or care for the young. It is the job of the workers to find food, feed the queen and care for the young. Without the workers the queen could not live and without the queen there would be no young.

Bumblebees are social insects. During spring a queen bumblebee nests and lays her eggs. The young hatch into workers— females that are smaller than the queen and are unable to breed. The workers take over the running of the nest. The queen is then free to produce more eggs, which are cared for by the workers. Toward the end of summer the queen lays eggs that hatch into male bumblebees and new queens. These offspring mate. The new queens leave the nest to find places to spend the winter. The original queen, males and workers will die when winter comes. When spring returns the young queens start their own colonies and the whole cycle begins again.

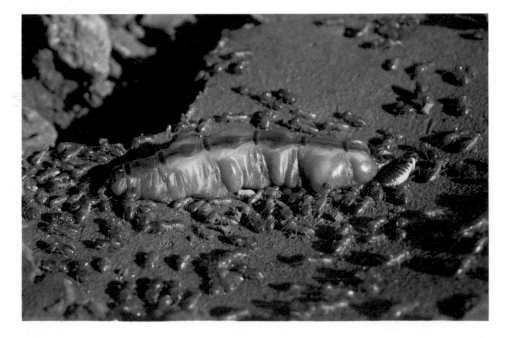

Termite king and queen
Termites live for a number of years. The queen and king spend all their lives together in a special chamber in the colony. After mating the queen becomes much larger than the king. Her body is swollen with eggs, and she can lay as many as 30,000 a day. Both queen and king are fed by the workers, who also tend the eggs and larvae. The queen's only job is to lay eggs, while the king's only job is to fertilize them.

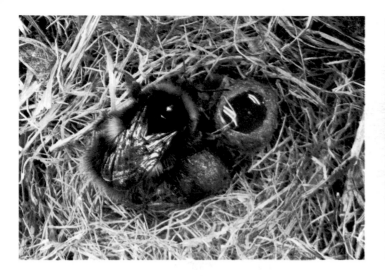

Queen bumblebee and nest

The old underground nests of mice and voles are often used by a queen bumblebee as a nest site. In the nest the queen builds a waxen egg chamber into which she lays about a dozen eggs. Before sealing the egg chamber she places in it a ball of pollen. Here the queen is brooding her egg chamber. Near to her is a full "honeypot" from which she will feed while she guards the nest.

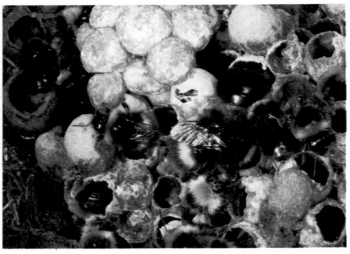

Worker bumblebees

The grub-like bumblebee larvae hatch, feed on the pollen inside the egg chamber, grow rapidly and then turn into pupae. After 20 days new adult workers emerge from these pupae. Their job is to find food and to care for the larvae that hatch after them. At the end of summer the queen lays a mixture of fertilized and unfertilized eggs. The larvae of the fertilized eggs are given extra food and grow into queens. The unfertilized eggs hatch into males. These young eventually mate and the new queens leave the colony.

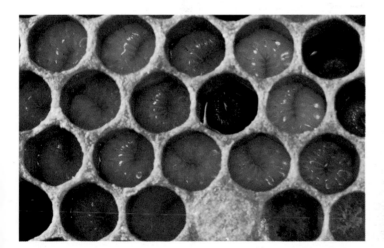

Developing honeybees

Queen honeybees live for about 3–5 years. During this time their only job is to lay eggs. Inside a beehive, eggs are laid in brood cells, like these, that are specially made by the workers. One egg is laid in each cell. The larvae hatch after 3–4 days and develop and change into pupae within their cells. After about three weeks they are ready to leave the cells as fully grown adults.

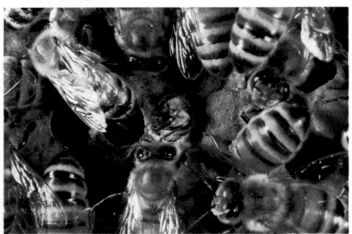

Honeybees hatching

The beehive is a very active place, containing one queen, several hundred males and thousands of female workers who are unable to breed. For the first three weeks after hatching the worker bees work in the hive, tending the eggs and young and repairing honey cells. Here you can see some workers watching over newly hatching bees. When a worker gets older her duties change and she flies off to the outside world, to collect and bring back pollen and nectar for the colony.

Nests

Some animals protect their eggs in a nest. In this shelter the eggs and young can be kept safely together. This makes it easier for the parent to look after the eggs and guard them from other animals. Birds are well known as nest builders, but some frogs, fish and other animals also build nests.

Nests come in many shapes and sizes and are made of many different materials. Birds' nests are often made from twigs, sticks, straw and other materials. These rough outer layers are then lined with a soft layer of fur, hair, moss or feathers. The soft lining helps to keep the eggs and young warm. Other animals like some frogs and fish make their nests from plants, small stones, or even air bubbles!

Many birds nest in trees and bushes, which provide a variety of well-hidden, safe places out of reach of most predators. One of the safest places is a hollow in a tree trunk. The entrance is often big enough to allow only the bird, and not other, larger, animals, to enter. But not all birds are tree-nesters. Seabirds nest on the narrow ledges of sea cliffs. Ducks, swans and other waterbirds nest on islands or among reeds where they are surrounded by water. Other birds may nest on the ground or under the ground and some even nest in buildings.

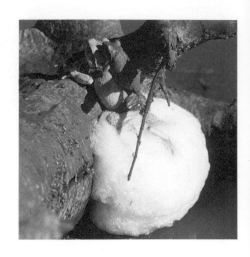

Foam-nesting frog
One of the strangest nests is that built by the foam-nesting frogs of tropical countries. In Africa these frogs live in trees and build their nests on leaves or branches that overhang fresh water. During mating the female sheds her eggs in a syrupy liquid, which both the male and female beat into a foam using their back legs. This forms a large frothy ball which hardens like a meringue around the newly laid eggs. The eggs hatch inside the ball and the young tadpoles grow in safety. They are kept moist within the foam and protected from harmful changes in temperature. After a few weeks the foam dissolves and the tadpoles fall into the water below.

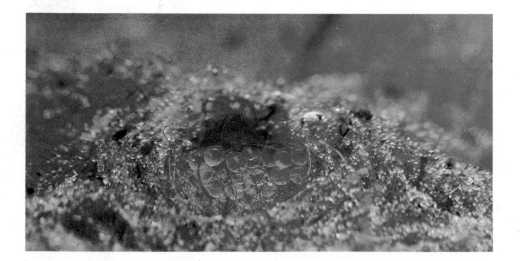

Stickleback's nest
The nest of the stickleback is found at the bottom of a river, stream or pond. Carefully made by the male fish out of fine weed and sand grains, it is about $1\frac{1}{2}$ in. in diameter. It is shaped so that the female can swim into and through it to lay her eggs. The male then follows to fertilize them.

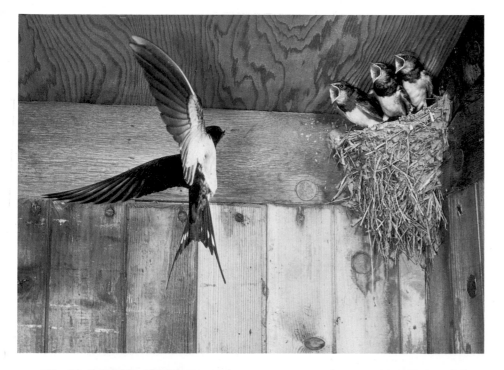

Swallow's nest

Swallows build their nests under the eaves of houses, stables and barns. The nest is made from tiny pellets of mud stuck together with spit and strengthened with pieces of straw. Only tiny amounts of mud can be collected in the parents' beaks at any one time, so it takes hundreds of journeys to finish the whole nest.

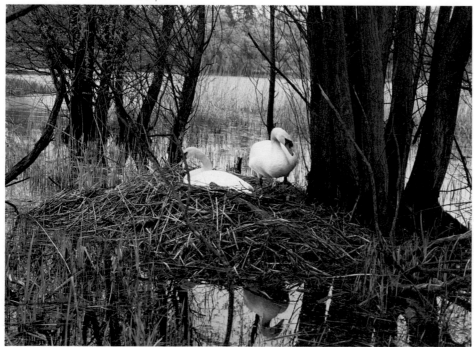

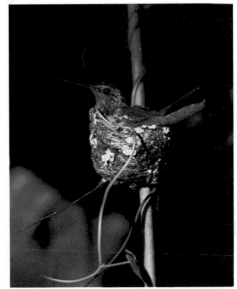

Swan's nest

The nest of these swans has been built among reeds at the edge of a lake or river. The nest is made of waterplants and twigs and is raised above water for safety. It is protected from land animals by the water around it. Its shape is roughly circular, with a dip in the center to stop the eggs from rolling out.

Hummingbird nest

Some of the smallest birds' nests are those built by hummingbirds. This nest of the emerald hummingbird from Trinidad is only 1 in. across and contains two eggs. It is cup-shaped and made of lichen, moss, hair and spiders' cobwebs. Built far out on a branch it is very difficult for predators to reach.

Incubation

Birds are warm-blooded and their eggs and young need to be kept warm while they grow. A bird's egg, if left alone, would quickly lose its heat and the growing young inside would die. For this reason birds "incubate," or sit on their eggs, using their own body warmth to brood them. The eggs of fish, amphibians and reptiles do not need any extra heat in order for the young to develop, although one or two snakes have special ways of keeping their eggs warm.

It is the parent bird's body touching the shell of the egg that warms it. During incubation some of the parent's belly feathers are shed, leaving a patch of naked skin called a "brood patch." This allows the body heat of the parent to pass directly to the egg. Pigeons and grebes shed some of their feathers naturally during incubation. Ducks and geese, however, have to pluck their feathers out to make a brood patch. These feathers are used to line the nest and to cover the eggs if the parent has to leave them.

The temperature at the top of the nest is warmer than at the bottom. So the parent regularly moves the eggs around and turns them over so they are warmed evenly. Pheasants turn their eggs once every hour, while a sparrow turns her eggs every 20 minutes. It is generally the female bird that incubates while the male brings her food, although with some birds like the dove, the male takes an equal turn in incubating.

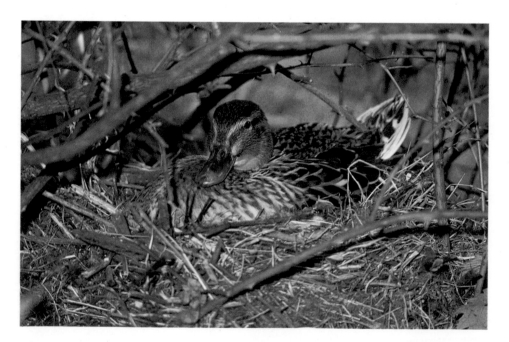

Mallard duck
Like this mallard duck, many female birds are dull in color compared to the brightly colored male. On the nest their coloring blends with their surroundings and by keeping very still they are difficult to see. The nest of the mallard is made of grass and dry leaves and lined with soft downy feathers which help to keep the eggs warm.

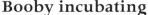

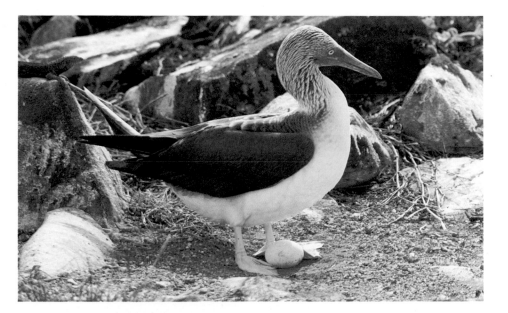

Booby incubating
This blue-footed booby lays only one egg which it incubates with its large webbed feet. Boobies have no brood patch, but the warm blood circulating through their feet provides the necessary heat. Gannets and some penguins also incubate their eggs with their feet.

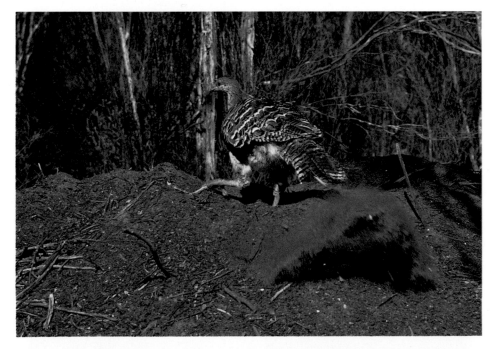

Mallee fowl
The mallee fowl of Australia does not incubate its eggs by brooding. Instead, male and female together dig a deep pit in the ground 2–3 yards across. They pile leaves and other matter into this until it is over a yard high. This vegetation slowly rots and gives off heat. When the right warmth is reached the female lays and buries her twenty or so eggs in the pit, which acts as an incubator. The male stays near the mound to test the temperature with his tongue. If it gets too hot he opens up the mound and if too cold he covers it over with more vegetation. After 7 weeks the young hatch, dig their way out and run away.

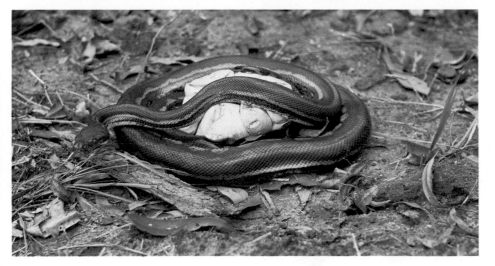

Python
The female python is one reptile that incubates her eggs. Wrapping herself tightly around them she keeps her eggs slightly warmer than the surrounding air. By doing this the young develop more quickly than other snakes' young. The female broods her eggs for two months, only leaving them for an occasional visit to water and, more rarely, to eat.

Eggs carried on the body

Some animals look after their eggs by taking them with them wherever they go. Attaching the eggs to their body in some way—on their back, front, or in a special pouch—means that the parent can lead a normal life while the eggs develop in safety. Some fish and frogs even brood their eggs in their mouths.

Animals have developed a variety of ways of carrying their eggs. Crayfish, lobsters and crabs attach their eggs to their belly or among the bristles of their legs. Wolf spiders and nursery web spiders lay their eggs in a cocoon of silk. This silken bundle is then attached to their body and away they go.

A few animals, like the female spiny anteater (see page 57), keep their eggs in special pouches on their body called brood pouches. The eggs and young are protected in the brood pouch while they develop. Some of the strangest kinds of brood pouches are those found on a few frogs and toads. During the breeding season these animals grow a special flap of skin on their back. The eggs develop under the flap until the young are ready to leave and look after themselves.

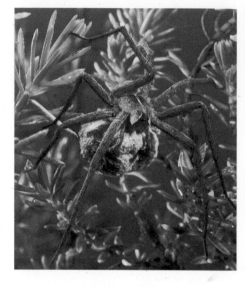

Nursery web spider
The 200–400 eggs of the nursery web spider are encased in a silken cocoon before being carried around by the female. She holds the cocoon in her jaws—it is so huge that it hangs underneath her. When hatching time is near the female makes a tent of leaves tied together with silk. Into this "nursery web" she hangs her egg sac and then sits on guard nearby. After hatching the spiderlings remain in the web for about a week before they go off on their own.

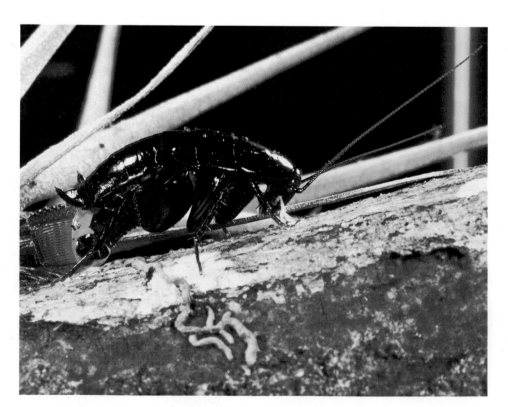

Cockroach
Cockroaches lay their eggs in a protective purse-like case. Most female cockroaches, like this one, carry the case sticking out from their rear end for only 2–3 days before dropping and burying it. One type of cockroach, however, carries the case until the young nymphs are ready to hatch, which could take 4–5 weeks. The nymphs are $\frac{1}{5}$ in. long when newly hatched and force the case to split open so they can wriggle free.

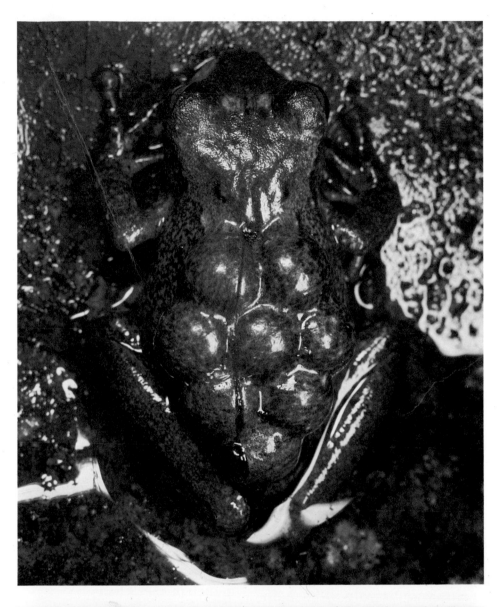

Marsupial frog
This female marsupial frog from South America has a brood pouch on her back. When she is ready to lay she raises her rear end and as her eggs are shed they roll down her back and through an opening into the pouch. Under the fold of skin the dozen or so eggs develop, and later hatch into tadpoles. When the fully developed young frogs are ready to leave, the female opens the split to the pouch with her back foot and they hop out.

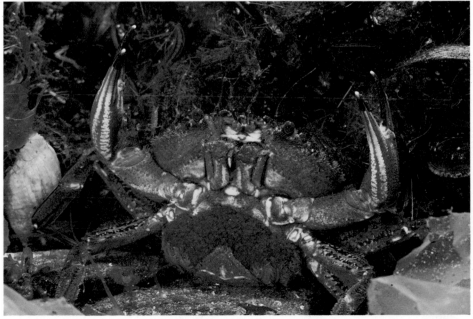

Crab in berry
During the breeding season female crabs develop a spongy skin on their belly. The eggs are laid and stuck onto this skin and held in place by the tail flap. Here the eggs develop and grow. Crabs are said to be "in berry" while carrying their eggs. Most crabs are able to keep their eggs moist as they live in or near water. Female ghost crabs live on land and every so often have to run into the water to wet their eggs.

Live birth

Mammal birth

Mammals are animals with hair or fur that feed their young on milk made in the mother's body. Mice, cats, deer, whales and humans are all mammals.

In nearly all mammals the baby animal develops in a special place inside the mother's body called the "womb." Inside the womb the baby is linked by a cord from its belly to a special organ on the wall of the womb called the "placenta." The placenta acts rather like a sieve. It allows food and oxygen from the mother's bloodstream to pass through the cord to the baby, and waste materials from the baby to pass out to the mother. It also prevents harmful matter from the mother reaching the baby. Inside the womb the baby can grow in warmth and safety.

The baby animal is enclosed in a sac of liquid. It twists and turns inside the sac as it grows. When the baby is ready to be born the muscles of the womb begin to tighten or "contract." These contracting muscles gradually push the baby out of the womb, down through the birth canal and out of the opening between the mother's legs. The fluid-filled sac bursts during the birth, and once outside, the baby animal begins to breathe. After the baby animal is born the placenta comes away from the wall of the womb and is pushed out of the mother's body. This is called the "afterbirth."

Not all mammal young develop in this way as you will see on page 42. Young mammals are very well cared for by their parents and have a much better chance of survival than the young of other animals. Because of this, mammals usually produce only a few young at a time.

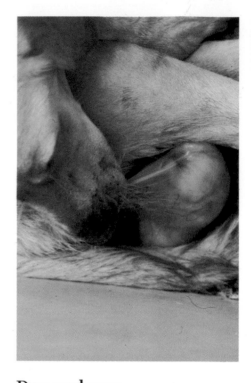

Dog and pup
After being born puppies are wet and covered with the remains of the sac. The mother will lick her pups clean before they start to suckle. The pups are blind at birth and keep warm by snuggling up to their mother's body.

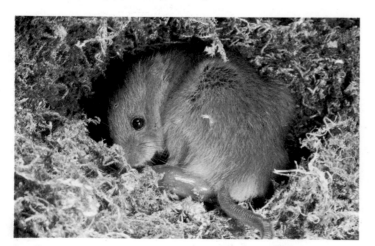

Harvest mouse
Baby harvest mice spend only 17–19 days in the womb before being born. The birth of the harvest mouse is very quick—this mother had five babies within 15 minutes. Each baby mouse is blind and naked. They need a lot of care from their mother before they can look after themselves.

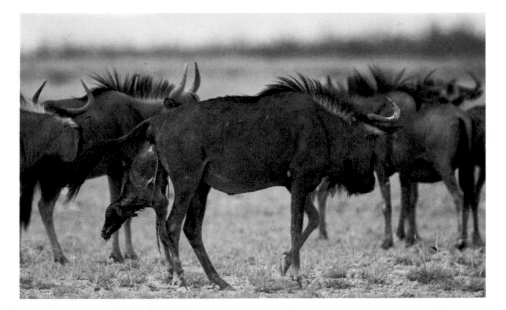

Wildebeest
While giving birth female wildebeests are often protected by a ring of females who will chase away any predators. The actual birth of the calf takes about an hour, and is a tiring process for both mother and young. Here the calf is being born and part of the sac that enclosed it while in the womb is still covering its body.

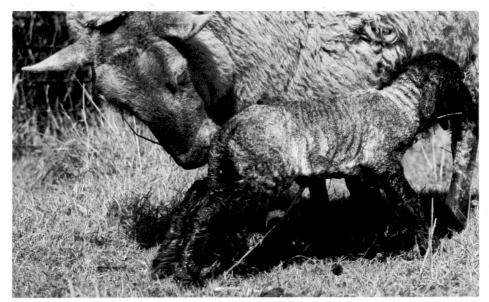

Lamb
Baby lambs spend nearly five months growing in the safety of the womb. Within minutes of being born, lambs can struggle to their feet and shakily stand and walk. Under this lamb's belly you can see the cord that joined it to the placenta in the womb. A few days after birth the cord will shrivel and fall off. Sheep generally give birth to one or two lambs a year.

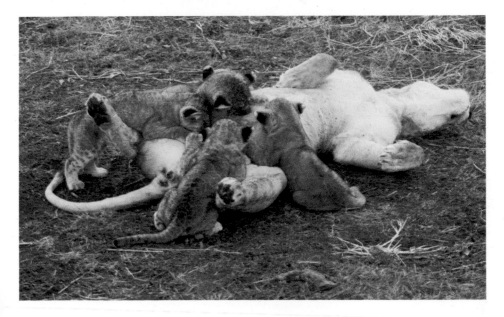

Lion cubs
Mammal babies, like these lion cubs, suckle their mother's milk soon after they are born. Milk is produced in special glands on the female's body and contains all the food a young mammal needs until it develops its first teeth and can eat other food.

Marsupial birth

Marsupials are a group of mammals whose young are born at a very early stage of development and usually complete their growth in a pouch on their mother's belly. These animals are found only in Australasia, South America and a few parts of North America. Koalas, kangaroos, wallabies and opossums are all marsupials.

Like other mammals, the baby marsupial begins to grow in the mother's womb, but there is no cord to join the mother to the baby while it develops. Instead the baby has a tiny yolk sac to provide it with food. The yolk does not last very long and the baby is born after only a short time in the womb—8 days for the small opossum and 33 days for the red kangaroo. At birth, the infant is rather wormlike, pink and hairless, with only its head and front limbs clearly developed. Newly born opossums are smaller than honeybees and in the largest kangaroo the newly born baby is only $\frac{3}{4}$ in. long.

When a female kangaroo is near to giving birth she cleans her pouch, holding it open with her forepaws and licking the inside. She also licks the fur in a line between her pouch and the opening of the birth canal, which is just under her tail. The tiny kangaroo baby is born head first. It grasps its mother's fur with its strong front legs and slowly climbs to the pouch following the line of licked fur. This journey takes about three minutes, and is absolutely vital for the baby. If it does not reach the pouch it will die. Once safely inside the pouch the baby searches for a nipple from which to feed.

Young opossums

Below left: Unlike kangaroos and koalas, which produce only one baby at a time, Virginia opossums give birth to several young— maybe as many as 12–14. Each youngster makes the dangerous journey to the pouch where it fastens onto one of the female's 13 nipples and starts to suckle. If more than 13 babies reach the pouch the last to arrive will starve and die as there are no more nipples. These young, at one month old, are naked, blind and helpless.

Below right: After 9 or 10 weeks in the pouch the young opossums are well developed and ready to leave. Still only about the size of a mouse, they climb onto their mother's back where they ride "piggyback" fashion, clinging tightly to her fur. It takes another three months for the young to become fully independent and to leave their mother.

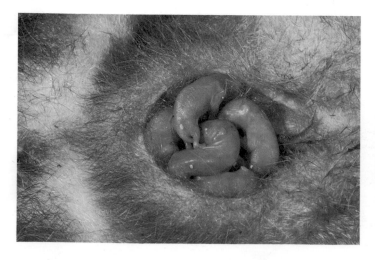

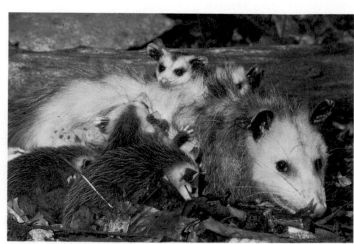

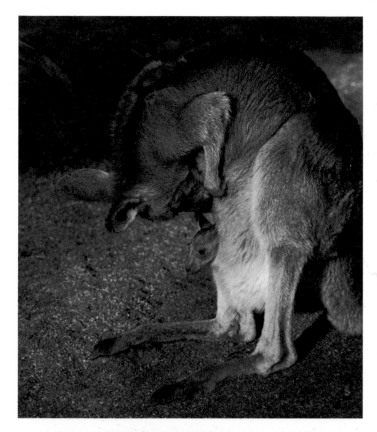

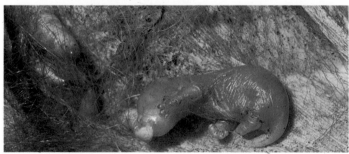

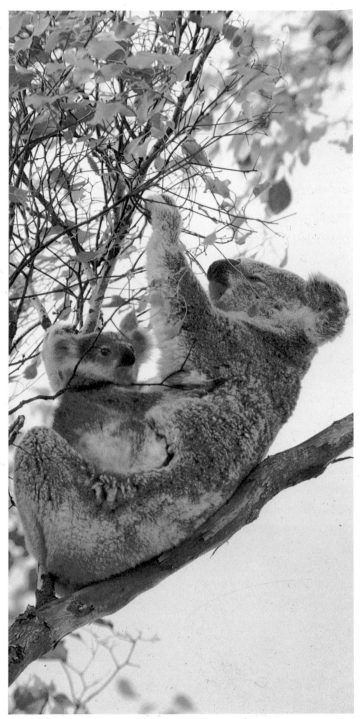

Young kangaroo in pouch

Inside the pouch of the female kangaroo are four nipples. The newly born baby fastens onto one of the nipples and starts to feed. The baby is completely helpless and over the next few months it grows rapidly. During this time the female will probably be suckling an older offspring, which returns to the pouch to feed from the same nipple it sucked from as a tiny baby. This nipple, as you can see, has now become swollen.

A young great gray kangaroo stays within its mother's pouch for about eight months. By this time it is fully formed and covered in fur. It is called a "joey." The joey then leaves the pouch and nibbles grass alongside its mother. For the next few months it returns to the safety of the pouch if danger threatens and still pushes its head in to feed now and again.

Koala and young

When the single young koala has left the pouch it rides on its mother's back or front. From here it has an excellent view of the food the adults eat and will reach out to pick the leaves of the eucalyptus tree in which the koalas live. When the youngster reaches half the adult weight it becomes too heavy to be carried and leaves the mother to climb about on its own.

Human birth

The human baby grows within its mother's womb for 40 weeks or about nine months. During this time, like all mammals, rapid growth and development takes place. Fertilization of the woman's egg takes place in one of her two "Fallopian tubes" or oviducts. From here the egg journeys down into her womb where it attaches itself to the soft lining and starts to grow.

Like other mammals the baby develops within a water-filled sac. The baby is joined to the placenta by a cord which carries food and oxygen to the baby and takes waste products away from it. The placenta grows with the developing baby for some weeks. Three weeks after fertilization the baby or embryo has developed a head and body. After two months the baby has all the parts of a fully formed human being, but these are not yet fully developed. At this stage the baby is called a "fetus" and is only $1\frac{1}{2}$ in. long.

By the end of the fifth month of pregnancy the fetus is 10 in. long—about half the length of the newborn baby. Inside the womb it moves, turning and kicking, and can hear the mother's heartbeats and all the sounds she makes talking, eating and drinking. About a month before birth most babies take up the birth position—generally with their head down toward the birth canal, although some babies are born feet first.

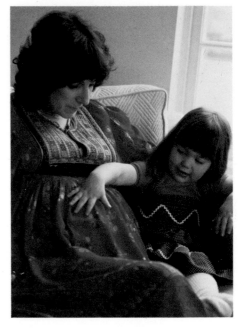

Pregnant woman
Generally by the fourth month of pregnancy the mother's abdomen begins to swell as the baby grows. When the baby begins to move inside the womb the mother can feel it, and the baby's movements can be seen and felt from the outside. By the end of nine months the mother's abdomen has become very large and the baby is ready to be born. The mother starts to feel the first of many contractions as the muscles of the womb tighten to push the baby out.

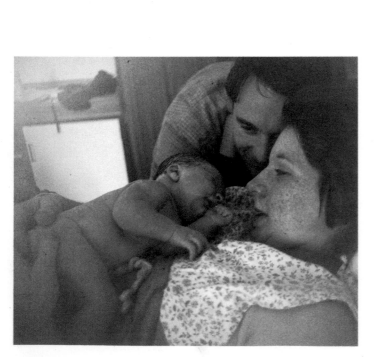

Birth
During birth the mother's contractions become stronger and more frequent. The baby is pushed out of the womb, down the birth canal to the opening between the mother's legs. Giving birth is exciting and very hard work and this mother is tired but very happy now that her baby is born. The cord, which still connects the baby to the placenta, is then tied and cut. The placenta now separates from the womb and is pushed out of the mother's body. A few days after birth the stub of the baby's cord shrivels and falls off. It leaves a scar on its tummy—the navel. The human baby depends on its parents for warmth, food and comfort, as it is unable to look after itself.

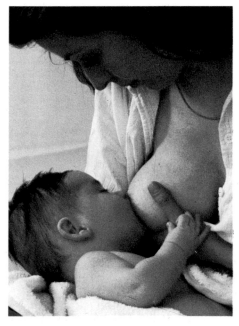

Suckling

Shortly after birth the baby begins to suckle. At first a special liquid called "colostrum" is produced in the mother's breasts, followed a few days later by milk. Human milk contains everything a baby needs for its first few months of life. As long as the baby feeds regularly from its mother, milk will be produced. When the baby stops being breast fed the mother's milk supply dries up. While the baby is feeding, the mother holds and cuddles it and this gives the baby a sense of security and comfort and a strong bond is built up between mother and child.

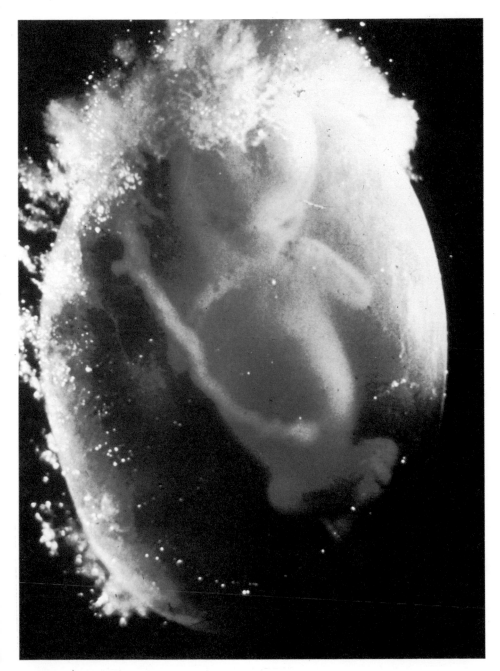

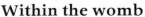

Within the womb

This picture is of the baby inside the mother's womb. The baby is enclosed in the water-filled sac where it is protected while it develops. It is nine weeks after the fertilization of the egg and the baby is fully formed. It has all its fingers, toes, ears, eyes and other parts, but will need to grow much bigger before it is born.

Other animals that give birth to live young

Mammals are not the only animals that give birth to fully formed young. A few fish, some snakes and lizards and other animals reproduce in this way too. These animals do not have a womb. Instead the fertilized egg generally develops within the female's oviduct. This acts as a living nest or incubator in which the young grow until they are ready to be born.

Each egg has a large supply of yolk on which the growing baby feeds. Instead of a shell, the egg is enclosed in a thin skin, which the young animal splits and struggles out of at birth. The young of these animals are born well developed and able to look after themselves. This is very important because there is often no parental care after birth.

All animals that give birth to live young produce only a small number of young at a time. Because the young are kept safe inside the female's body while they are growing, they have a much better chance of surviving than the young that hatch from eggs laid outside the body.

Timber rattlesnake
The female timber rattlesnake has one, sometimes two, litters of young a year. There may be between 10 and 20 young in each litter. Soon after each baby is born it struggles out of the skin that surrounded it inside the mother's oviduct. For a while the young snakes may stay near the mother but eventually they move off into the undergrowth to start life on their own.

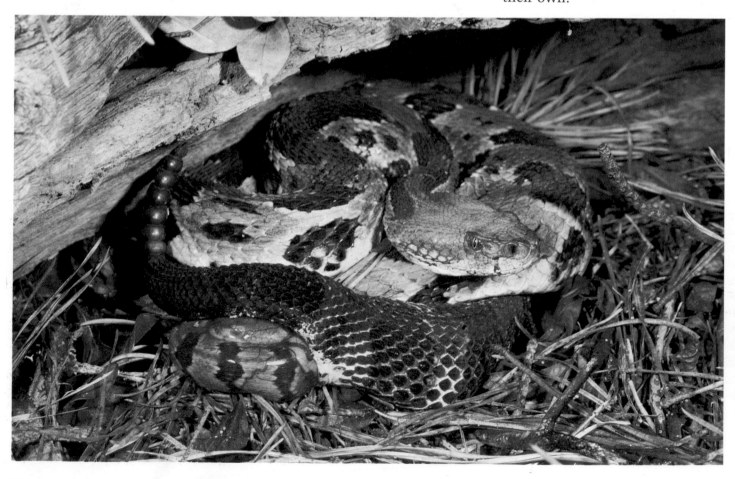

Anemone

Beadlet anemones, like this one, are found almost all over the world in rock pools on the sea-shore. This type of anemone gives birth to fully formed young and does not shed its eggs and sperm into the water. The fertilized eggs develop within the adult's body. At birth the young are released through the anemone's only body opening—the mouth.

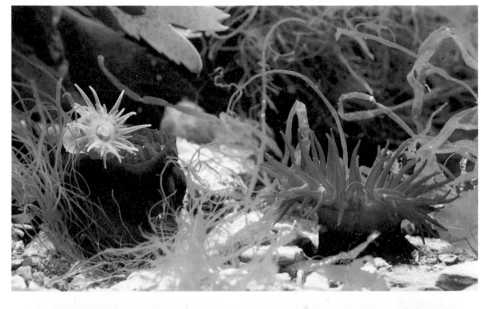

Guppies

Guppies are freshwater fish that are found in South America and the West Indies. The pregnant female guppy starts to look quite big and fat as the time for birth approaches. Her fertilized eggs are kept inside her until the young are well developed and ready to be born. As soon as the young are born they swim away to lead an independent life. If they stay too long near their mother they may be eaten!

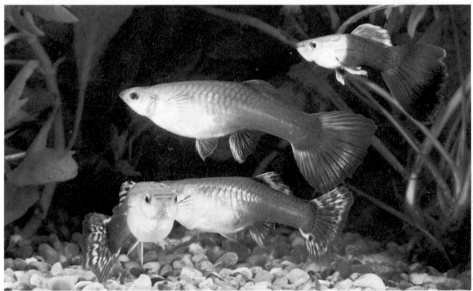

Aphid

During summer when there is plenty of food available, female aphids are able to give birth without mating. The young look exactly like their mother only smaller. Each one is independent from birth and can produce its own young within 8–10 days, so their numbers increase rapidly. As autumn approaches, aphids mate and lay eggs. The eggs survive through the winter to hatch in the spring.

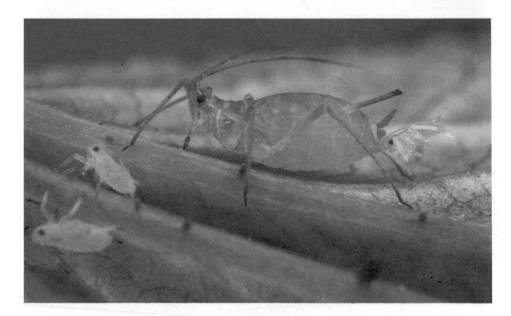

Parental care

Parental care of young animals

Although many animals abandon their eggs and young, a number of creatures continue to care for their young after they are born or hatched. Some spiders, insects, frogs and reptiles, as well as mammals and birds, all care for their young.

Young animals are very likely to fall prey to enemies. They are not so strong as their parents and cannot move so quickly. They are also inexperienced and have yet to discover how to protect themselves. Those animals which lay a small number of eggs, or give birth to only a few young, need to take more care of them to make sure that some survive. The weeks or months of parental care give the young time to grow stronger, until eventually they are able to look after themselves. During this time the parent may put its own life at risk to defend its young. If it is killed, but the young survive, then the animal has succeeded in its task of parental care.

Parental care may be shared by both parents, each taking a part in looking after their growing young, as many birds and mammals do. Some animals leave the care to the father as you will see on page 50, while crocodiles, some frogs, spiders and many mammals leave the care to the mother.

The female crocodile is a caring mother. Although she buries her 40 or more eggs underground, she remains nearby to guard them. When the young crocodiles are ready to hatch they start to chirp. These sounds are so loud that they can be heard by the female on guard duty nearby. She digs away the sand to help her young emerge and gently picks them up in her mouth and takes them to a quiet nursery pool.

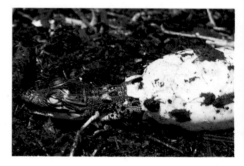

Crocodile
As the young crocodiles, each about 4 in. long, struggle out of their shells the female picks them up in her mouth. She has a special pocket in the bottom of her mouth where she can hold about six young at a time. Carrying a mouthful, the female takes her young to the nursery pool before returning to pick up more. The young that hatch while the female is away have no protection and may well be killed and eaten by hungry birds or other creatures. She remains with her young in the nursery pool for a few months and during this time she chases away any strangers. Eventually the young crocodiles venture away from the nursery pool to look after themselves.

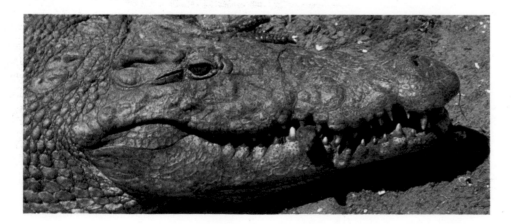

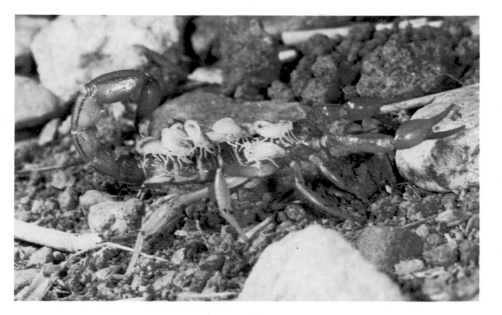

Scorpion

Female scorpions keep their fertilized eggs inside them until they hatch. The babies then crawl out and climb onto their mother's back, where they stay for about two weeks, safely protected by the female's deadly sting! After their first molt the young are ready to care for themselves.

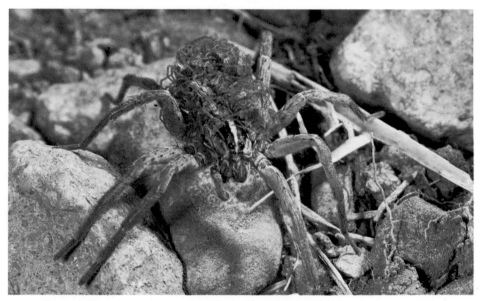

Wolf spider

The female wolf spider lays her eggs in a cocoon which she attaches to her abdomen and takes with her wherever she goes. When the tiny spiderlings hatch they climb onto her back and cling to her hairy body. For the next couple of weeks the young are able to grow stronger while being carried around by the female. After this, they go off on their own and look after themselves.

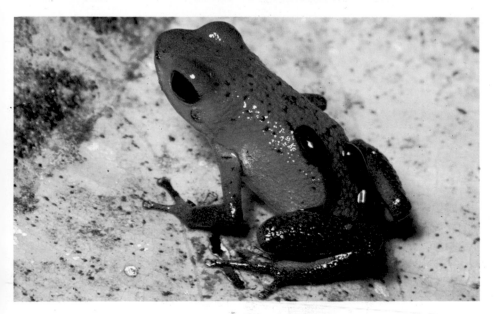

Poison dart frog

Poison dart frogs live in the rain forests of Central America. The female lays about 15 eggs on the ground where they are guarded by one of the parents. After about 10 days the tadpoles hatch and climb onto the female's back where they stick to her moist skin. In this way they are carried to pools of water trapped among the leaves of large plants. Each tadpole slides off the female's back into its own pool where it grows into an adult frog.

Fathercare

The important job of caring for the eggs and young is some-times done by the male. The female is then free to feed and build up her strength before finding a new mate and laying more eggs. Several animals, including some fish, frogs, toads, insects and birds leave the care of the young to the father.

These fathers look after their young in many different ways. Some birds and fishes build nests, while others may carry their eggs on their backs or wrapped around their legs. The king penguin incubates his solitary egg on his feet during the Antarctic winter, while the male emu incubates a clutch of 8–10 eggs in a large nest on the ground. After the emu chicks have hatched the father guards them for 18 months until they are able to look after themselves. Other males, like the seahorse, keep their young safe within a brood pouch.

A few male frogs and fish have a very strange way of caring for the young: they keep them in their mouths As long as the father does not eat or swallow, the young are safe from danger. While in his mouth the eggs and young are jostled around. This bumping and rubbing keeps them clean of mold that could kill them. Mouth-brooding is a very safe and successful way of caring for both eggs and young.

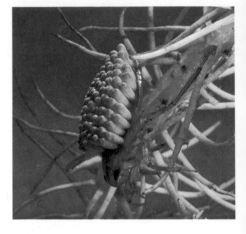

Water bug
The male water bug may be a reluctant egg-minder, as the female forcibly attaches her eggs to his back with a waterproof glue. Then the female leaves and the male carries the eggs with him, where-ever he goes, until the young hatch about a month later.

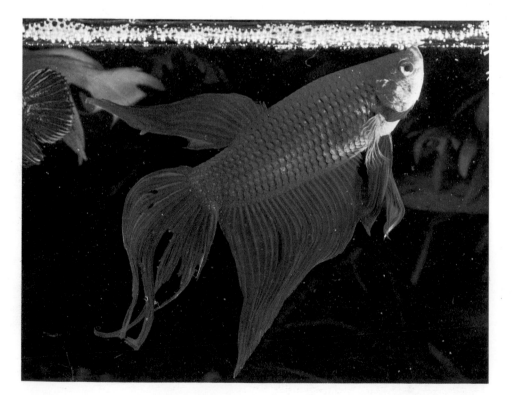

Siamese fighting fish
This floating nest of bubbles has been made by the male Siamese fighting fish for his eggs and young. He sucks air into his mouth and then blows out a stream of bubbles which he coats in a slimy substance. This substance makes the bubbles stick together and stops them from bursting. He continues to do this until a nest about an inch wide and $\frac{1}{2}$ in. thick is formed. After mating, the male catches the eggs in his mouth before they sink and blows them into the nest. He watches over the eggs, and later guards the young until they are ready to swim away.

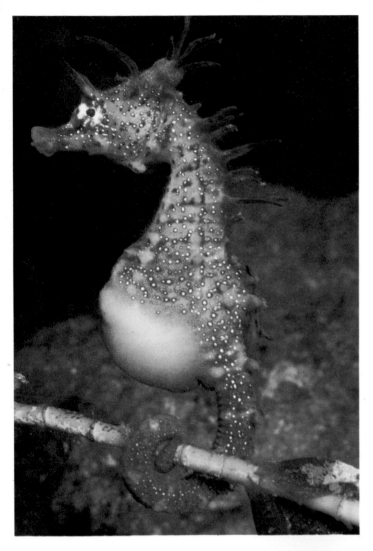

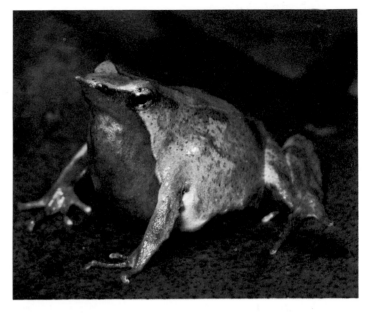

Darwin's frog

The male Darwin's frog from South America keeps his young in his mouth for safety. The eggs from several females are laid on the ground and then guarded by a group of males. When the eggs are about to hatch each male scoops up about seventeen with his tongue and swallows them. The eggs slide into his swollen vocal sac where they hatch and here the young grow into tiny frogs. When they are ready to leave, the male gulps several times, suddenly yawns, and out of his mouth jump the froglets.

Seahorse

The male seahorse cares for the eggs after they are fertilized. He keeps them in a pouch on his belly where they develop. He can carry as many as 200 eggs, which take 4–5 weeks to hatch. When the young are ready to be born, the male anchors himself by winding his tail around a firm object. He then bends and straightens his body in a series of jerks until a baby seahorse shoots out from the opening of the pouch. The young seahorses look just like their parents, but are only $\frac{1}{25}$ in. long.

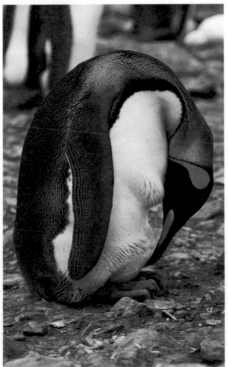

King penguin

King penguins breed in large colonies on islands in the cold Antarctic ocean. After mating and egg-laying the female passes the single egg to the male. He balances it on his feet and covers it with a fold of belly skin to keep it warm. The female then leaves for the sea to feed and build up her strength. The male spends the next $7\frac{1}{2}$ weeks incubating the egg. When the chick is ready to hatch the female returns. The male is then free to go off to feed at sea after his long starvation. When he returns both male and female take turns fetching food for the chick.

The care and protection of young birds

Young birds hatch out of their eggs at varying stages of development. Some like the young of pelicans, woodpeckers, robins and blackbirds, hatch blind, naked and helpless. These young need a lot of care from their parents. They need to be kept warm until their feathers grow and to be fed by their parents until they are old enough to find their own food.

Other birds, like the young of ducks, hens and pheasants hatch at a well-developed stage and are active immediately. They have their eyes open and are covered in thick down which helps to keep them warm. Many of these young hatch in nests on the ground and it is important for them to be able to move quickly to escape from danger. Young ducks, swans and other waterbirds have to be able to swim immediately as they live and feed in water. Such well developed young are usually able to feed themselves. They will peck and scratch at anything that looks like food and soon learn what is good to eat. Occasionally the mother will point with her beak to suitable food to encourage her young to try the food for themselves.

There are some downy chicks, however, that are fed by their parents to begin with. The chicks of gulls are sturdy and are able to leave the nest shortly after hatching, but they cannot fly in search of food. Instead the parent feeds them on returning home from a fishing trip. When the chicks are older they will fly off and practice catching their own fish.

Sparrowhawk young
Young birds of prey, like these sparrowhawks, hatch with a thin covering of down and with their eyes open, but they are quite helpless and rely on their parents for food and warmth. The nests of these birds are high in trees away from danger. The parents bring freshly killed meat to the nest for the young, and then tear off strips small enough for the chicks to swallow. Like most other birds, the young are born at a time of year when there is plenty of food available.

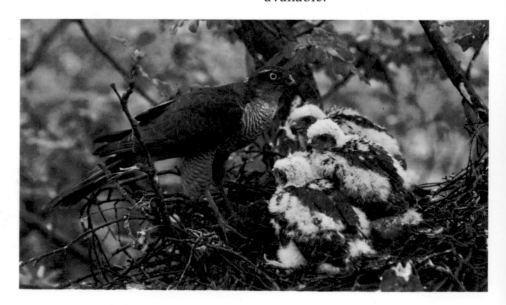

Naked nestlings

These naked nestlings of the hedgesparrow have no control over their body heat. They rely on their parents for warmth until their own feathers grow. The parent will brood the chicks to keep them warm. As soon as their eyes are open the young become much more active, chirping and stretching their wings in preparation for flying and leaving the nest.

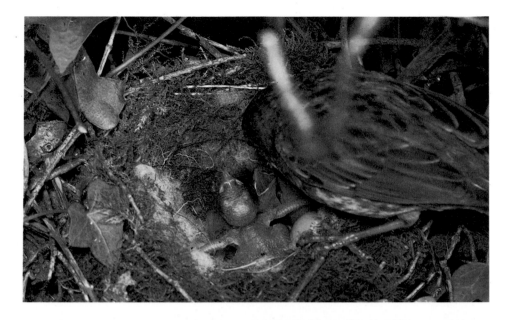

Young robins

Although now fully feathered, these young robins still gape for food. They are entirely dependent on their parents while in the nest. As the parent lands on the edge of the nest to feed them, the young feel the jolt and open their mouths. The bright markings in and around the nestlings' mouths encourage the parent to feed them. After the young have left the nest they may still be fed for many weeks by their parents until they become independent.

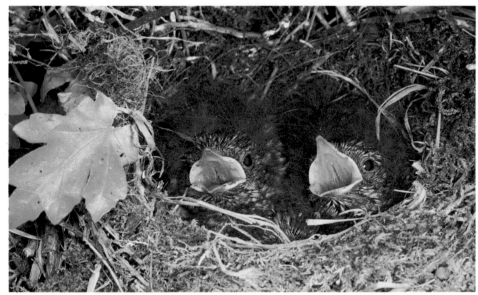

Mallard ducklings

These mallard ducklings have been led by their mother to an area rich in food. Here they have to discover for themselves what is good to eat. They will hunt and eat grubs, worms, insects, small frogs and fish, as well as feeding on waterplants and seeds. If the ducklings are well fed they can keep warm all day. At night and in bad weather they huddle together for warmth, or seek shelter among their parents' feathers.

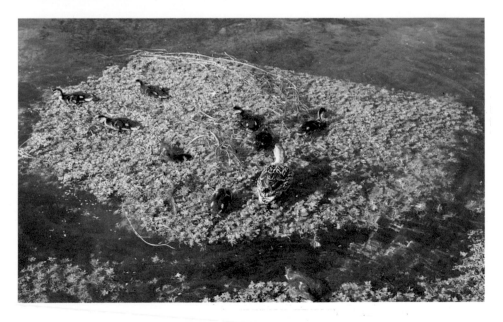

The care and protection of young birds
continued

Most birds continue to care for their young until they are well able to look after themselves. For small songbirds, this is quite a short time and may allow the parents to raise two or even three broods a year. Larger birds take longer to raise their young and may have only one brood a year. The large wandering albatross rears one chick every two years—each chick spending almost a year in the nest, being fed and cared for by its parents.

The parents not only provide food and keep the chicks warm— they also protect their young from danger. Larger birds like swans and geese fight off any enemies with their wings and beaks. Terns and other birds that live in colonies gang up and dive-bomb any intruders into their nesting colony. Some birds carry their young away from danger. Red-tailed hawks gently pick up their chicks with their powerful talons and fly off, while the woodcock picks its youngsters up and carries them away between its thighs.

Many birds are able to warn their young of danger by special alarm calls. The chicks react immediately by keeping very still and quiet. They will start to move again only after the parents have given the "all clear."

Canada goose
Water birds, like this Canada goose, often allow their young to ride on their back. Not only does it keep the chicks warm among the parent's feathers, but it also keeps them safe. On water the chicks have quite a struggle to keep up with their parents and may be in danger of being pulled under and eaten by eels, pike or other predators.

Blacksmith plover
A common trick used by ground-nesting birds is to lure intruders away from their young. This blacksmith plover pretends to be injured to attract the young elephant's attention. Dragging her wing, she leads the inquisitive elephant a safe distance away from her nest. She will then fly back to her chicks which have remained undiscovered.

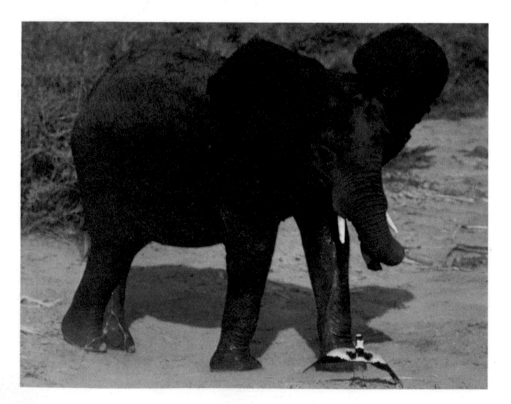

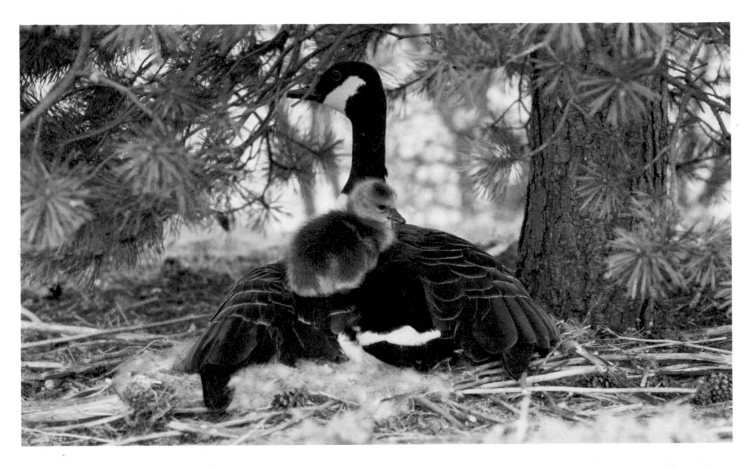

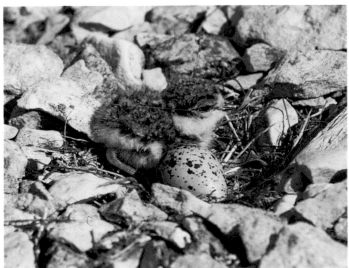

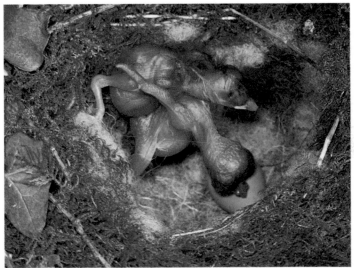

Plover chick

The eggs and chicks of many ground-nesting birds, like this plover chick, blend in well with their background. The chicks' coloring of brown, black and yellow speckles matches a wide range of natural objects around them. They are very difficult to see, especially if they keep still and quiet. This camouflage is essential for their survival, when there is nowhere for them to hide.

Young cuckoo

Cuckoos do not build their own nests but lay their eggs in the nests of other birds. The young cuckoo generally hatches first and moves to the bottom of the nest. It then balances each remaining egg, or newly hatched young, on its back and throws it out of the nest. In this picture the young cuckoo is throwing out a baby hedgesparrow. When on its own in the nest it receives constant attention from its foster parents and grows rapidly, until it becomes almost too big for the nest.

Helpless mammal young

Many mammals give birth to blind and naked young that need to be looked after for some time before they can fend for themselves. Generally the young of these animals develop in their mother's womb for quite a short time—lions and tigers give birth after about four months, foxes after 7–8 weeks, while the young of some mice are born after only 2–3 weeks.

Such youngsters are usually born into a safe, warm nest, burrow or other shelter where the female can care for them. The naked young need to be kept warm until they grow their own fur. The mother never leaves them for long, as they need to suckle regularly on her milk. When their eyes have opened, which takes about 6 days for lion cubs, 10 days for house mice and 14 days for tiger cubs, the young become more active and playful.

Small mammals, like mice and voles, grow and leave the nest quickly. Young house mice are able to look after themselves three weeks after birth, and these mammals may have as many as five litters a year. The helpless young of larger mammals such as lions and tigers spend much longer, maybe some months, in their nest or den. Even when the cubs have left this shelter and have stopped being suckled, they need to stay with their mother for several months. During this time they are taught how to hunt for food and look after themselves before becoming independent.

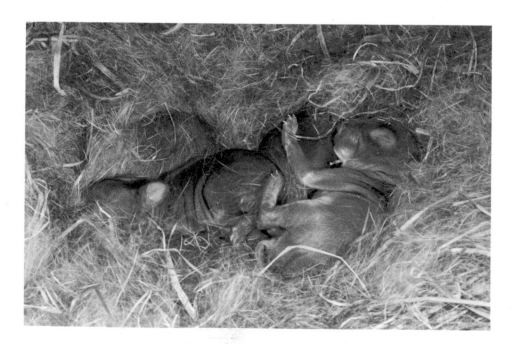

Rabbits
The female rabbit gives birth to 3–6 young in a warm, underground burrow. The nest is lined with grass, straw and fur from her own body. At birth each kitten, as it is called, weighs less than 2 oz. The female leaves her babies in the nest and goes off to feed, returning once a day to suckle them. After each visit she covers the entrance with earth to hide it and also to keep the nest warm. The young rabbits grow quickly and at 3 weeks old start to explore the outside world.

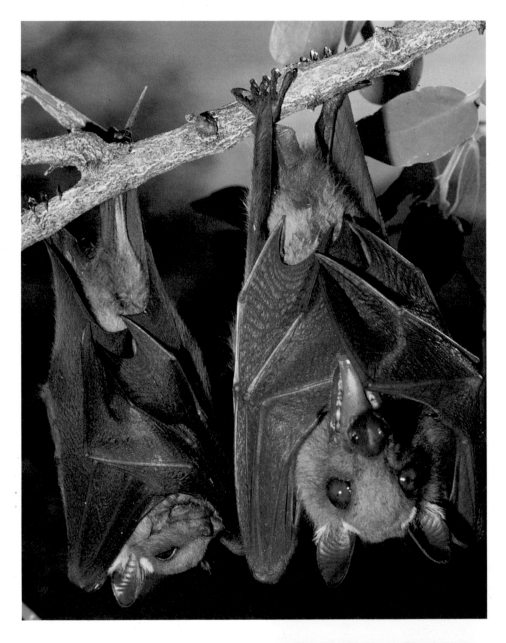

Fruit bats

Bats give birth about 2 months after mating. The baby is very small, blind and naked and the mother takes it with her wherever she flies, with the baby clinging to her fur. When the youngster has grown too heavy to be carried, the mother leaves it hanging in the roost while she goes off to hunt. She returns regularly to suckle the baby and hangs next to it while sleeping during the day. At 4 months a young bat is fully grown, but does not yet have its adult fur. Bats usually have only one baby a year.

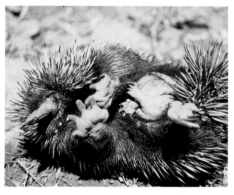

Spiny anteater

The spiny anteater and the duck-billed platypus are very unusual mammals as they lay eggs. The female anteater lays one or two soft-shelled eggs directly into a pouch on her belly. The young hatch after 7–10 days and remain in the pouch for about seven weeks, feeding on milk from the mother. When their spines start to grow and they are too big to remain in the pouch, the mother scoops them out. She keeps them warm in a nest until they are old enough to care for themselves.

Harvest mouse

Harvest mice weave their nests in grainfields or tall grass well above the ground. In the soft, cozy home the 3–8 babies remain safe and warm until they make their first journey outside, about 15 days after they are born. The mother guards her young carefully. If she is disturbed, or danger threatens, she removes her babies to a new home which she has prepared. She carries them in her mouth, one by one, until they are all safe. Other animals, such as cats and lions also remove their young to a new place if disturbed.

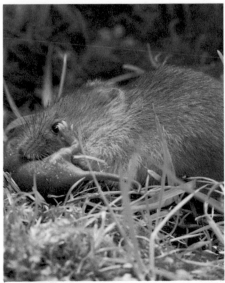

Mammal young born ready for action

Not all mammals give birth to helpless youngsters. Hares, deer, elephants and whales are some of the many mammals whose young are well developed, alert and ready for action as soon as they are born. These young generally develop within their mother's womb for quite a long time. Horses give birth after eleven months, and the elephant carries her baby for almost two years. Although they are dependent on their mother for milk, many of these youngsters are also able to eat plants and other foods right after birth. They may continue to suckle from their mother for some time—up to a year for the moose and 3–4 years for young elephants.

Whales, dolphins and porpoises are mammals that have become fully adapted to living in water. Their young grow for about a year in the mother's womb before being born underwater. The single whale baby is born tail first so that it can receive oxygen from its mother until the very last moment of birth. As soon as the calf is born it is lifted to the water's surface by the mother so that it can take its first breath of air. The baby can swim right after birth and will suckle from its mother for about a year.

Springbok
Springbok are found in South Africa, and like many of the African herd animals are continually on the move across the grassy plains in search of food. The young are born while the parents are traveling and must be able to move with the herd as soon as possible. The herd is always at risk from meat-eating animals like lions, who will pick out any weaklings such as the newly born. This calf, very recently born, has risen shakily to its feet and will be ready to move with the herd in a few hours' time.

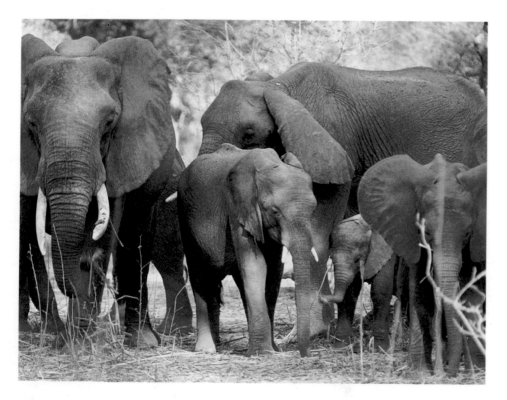

Elephants
Female African elephants live together in a group while the males live apart in separate herds. A female elephant is accompanied by other females when she gives birth and they stay with her until the baby is able to follow its mother. These females are quick to defend the mother and baby if danger threatens. A few hours after birth the baby is ready to follow the group. If the baby becomes tired while following, it will hang onto its mother's tail, with its trunk, to help it along.

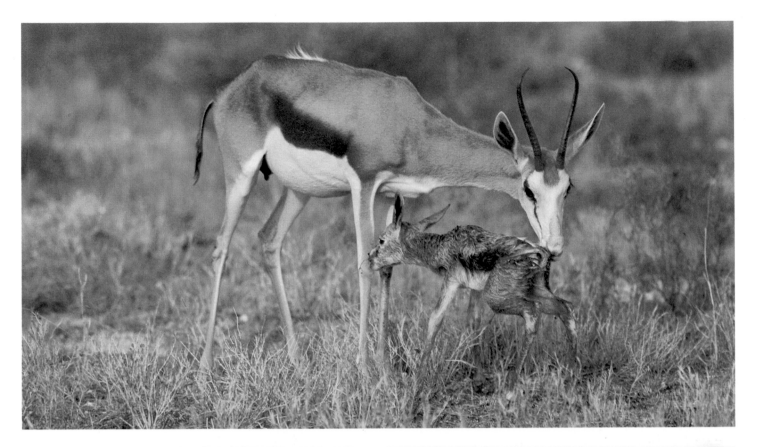

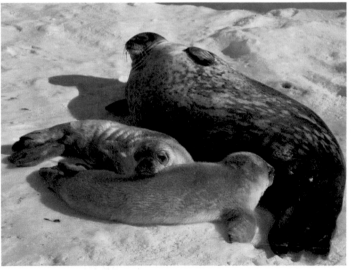

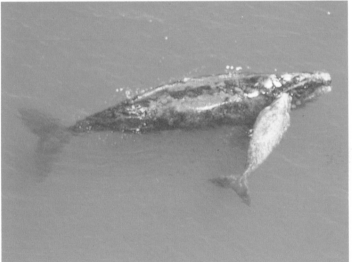

Seals

Seal pups, like these Weddell seal twins, are born on land but have to learn to live in water shortly after birth. They are well developed but rather thin when born. The pup feeds on its mother's rich milk and quickly builds up a thick layer of fat under its skin. This helps to keep it warm and also to float easily in water.

Whales

Like all mammals this southern right whale calf, seen from the air with its mother, is fed on mother's milk. The baby feeds underwater every few minutes between trips to the surface for breathing. The mother's nipples are on the underside of her belly and when the calf wants to suckle it takes one into its mouth. The mother then squirts the milk into the calf's mouth. This helps the calf to get a lot of milk in a very short time.

Learning about life

Many baby mammals spend a long time with their parents learning about life before they leave to look after themselves. Being taught how to hunt for food, live with other members of the group, defend themselves against enemies and later look after their own young are all very important lessons. Without these valuable months or years of teaching, the young animals would not be able to survive as adults.

Young animals need to be able to keep up with their parents if they are to survive and learn. Many females, like the chimpanzee and opossum, carry their young piggy-back style. Even in the water, walrus and hippos allow their young to ride on their backs if tired. The young are kept safe by being carried in this way. They are also able to watch their parents closely and to learn which foods are good to eat and where to find them, as well as many other things.

Playing is very important as it teaches the young many skills. Young lions and tigers stalk and pounce on each other in pretend hunts and fights. As well as learning how to test their strength against each other the young exercise and develop their muscles in readiness for the real fights and struggles of adult life.

Young monkeys also learn by playing, watching and copying their parents and other members of the group. These youngsters soon learn the many different gestures and calls of the adults that tell them about danger, fear, friendliness and aggression. Eventually, if no disaster befalls them, the young monkey becomes an adult and finds its own place within the group.

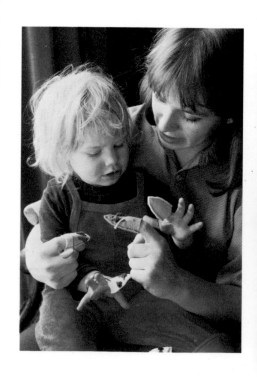

Young child
As a young child grows it learns to talk. Speech opens up a whole new world to the infant. As soon as it can speak it can communicate more easily with other people and never stops discovering about life. The length of time a human child is dependent on its parents is the longest of any animal, lasting for many years.

Baboons

These baboons learn about child-rearing by watching other females give birth and care for their young. Babies are cared for mostly by the mother, but at times other members of the group, including the males, nurse, groom, fuss over and protect the young. During the first few years of life the young baboon stays close to its mother. It learns a great deal from her and also from playing with its brothers, sisters and cousins.

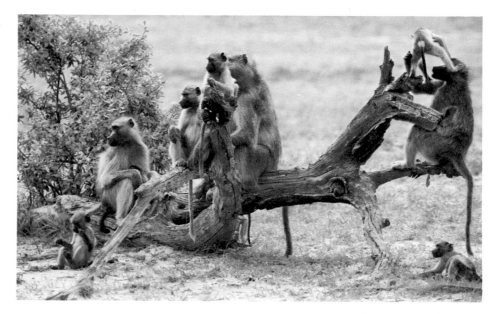

Lioness and cubs

When they are about three months old lion cubs get their first lessons in hunting, staying hidden while they watch the adult females make a kill. Once the lion has fed, the mother calls her cubs to come and feed. When three-quarters grown they begin to take a more active role in hunting, helping to confuse the prey and stop it escaping from the lionesses. Only when fully grown will the cubs have the speed and strength to make a kill of their own.

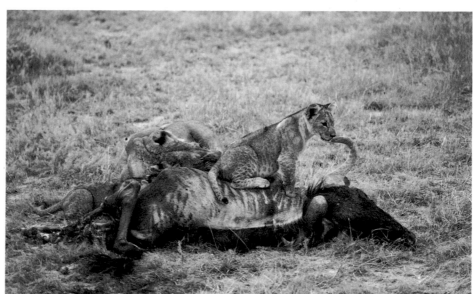

Grizzly bear cubs

Grizzly bears give birth to two or three cubs in a warm, hidden den. After two months the cubs are strong enough to follow their mother and they leave the den in search of food. The cubs are taught to hunt for berries, roots and small animals and they also learn to catch fish in the fast flowing rivers of northern America. After six months or so the young bears are well equipped to strike out on their own.

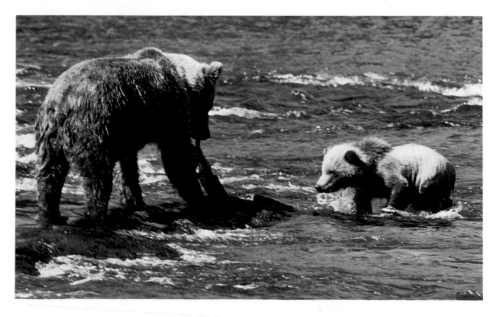

Index

Figures in bold type indicate the page where the entry is defined.

Acknowledgments

All photographs are copyright © Oxford Scientific Films unless otherwise stated. Photographers are listed starting with the picture at top left.

Page 8 Sean Morris
Page 9 Peter Parks: John Cheverton: Peter Parks
Page 10 Peter Parks
Page 11 Gene Cox: Michael Fogden: J. A. L. Cooke
Page 12 Doug Allan: G. I. Bernard
Page 13 G. I. Bernard: G. I. Bernard: J. A. L. Cooke
Page 14 Peter Parks
Page 15 G. I. Bernard: G. I. Bernard: Z. Leszczynski © Animals Animals/OSF
Page 16 G. I. Bernard: G. I. Bernard
Page 17 Peter Parks: Peter Parks: J. A. L. Cooke
Page 18 Peter Parks: Peter Parks
Page 19 G. I. Bernard: Peter Parks: David Thompson
Page 20 J. A. L. Cooke
Page 21 J. A. L. Cooke: J. A. L. Cooke: J. A. L. Cooke: G. I. Bernard
Page 22 Peter Parks
Page 23 Peter Parks: David Shale: Z. Leszczynski © Animals Animals/OSF
Page 24 G. I. Bernard: G. I. Bernard
Page 25 J. A. L. Cooke: J. A. L. Cooke: G. I. Bernard
Page 26 J. A. L. Cooke
Page 27 Maurice Tibbles: J. A. L. Cooke: G. I. Bernard
Page 28 G. I. Bernard: J. A. L. Cooke
Page 29 G. I. Bernard: J. S. and E. J. Woolmer: J. A. L. Cooke
Page 30 G. I. Bernard: F. H. Wylie © Frank Lane Agency

Page 31 J. A. L. Cooke: J. A. L. Cooke: Dennis Green © Survival Anglia Ltd/OSF
Page 32 N. Mark Collins
Page 33 D. M. Shale: D. M. Shale: David Thompson: David Thompson
Page 34 Robin Buxton: David Thompson
Page 35 Stephen Dalton: Helen Price: J. A. L. Cooke
Page 36 David Thompson
Page 37 C. M. Perrins: Jen and Des Bartlett © Survival Anglia Ltd/OSF: © Bruce Coleman Ltd
Page 38 J. A. L. Cooke: J. A. L. Cooke
Page 39 G. I. Bernard: G. I. Bernard
Page 40 © Camilla Jessel FRPS: Sean Morris
Page 41 Jen and Des Bartlett © Survival Anglia Ltd/OSF: G. I. Bernard: David Cayless
Page 42 Breck P. Kent © Animals Animals/OSF: E. R. Degginger © Animals Animals/OSF
Page 43 M. Austerman © Animals Animals/OSF: Alan Root © Survival Anglia Ltd/OSF: Jen and Des Bartlett © Survival Anglia Ltd/OSF
Page 44 © Anthea Sieveking/Vision International: © Camilla Jessel FRPS
Page 45 © CNRI/Vision International: © Anthea Sieveking/Vision International
Page 46 Z. Leszczynski © Animals Animals/OSF
Page 47 G. I. Bernard: G. H. Thompson: G. I. Bernard
Page 48 David Curl: John Visser © Bruce Coleman Ltd
Page 49 J. A. L. Cooke: J. A. L. Cooke: Michael Fogden

Page 50 J. A. L. Cooke: G. H. Thompson
Page 51 Rudie H. Kuiter: Michael Fogden: Cindy Buxton and Annie Price © Survival Anglia Ltd/OSF
Page 52 Chris Knights © Survival Anglia Ltd/OSF
Page 53 J. A. L. Cooke: G. I. Bernard: M. J. Bailey
Page 54 David Cayless
Page 55 G. I. Bernard: Ted Levin © Animals Animals/OSF: J. A. L. Cooke
Page 56 G. I. Bernard
Page 57 P. and W. Ward: Jen and Des Bartlett © Survival Anglia Ltd/OSF: G. I. Bernard
Page 58 G. I. Bernard
Page 59 Jen and Des Bartlett © Survival Anglia Ltd/OSF: Doug Allan: Jen and Des Bartlett © Survival Anglia Ltd/OSF
Page 60 © Anthea Sieveking/ Vision International
Page 61 G. I. Bernard: Donn Renn: Brian Milne © Animals Animals/OSF

Front cover © Hugo van Lawick